Guide to the Primary Care Guidelines

Fourth Edition

Guide to the Primary Care Guidelines

Fourth Edition

Edited by

Dr Peter Smith OBE
General Practitioner, Kingston upon Thames
President, National Association of Primary Care

Foreword by
Dr David Colin-Thomé OBE
National Clinical Director for Primary Care

Radcliffe Publishing
Oxford • New York

Radcliffe Publishing Ltd
18 Marcham Road
Abingdon
Oxon OX14 1AA
United Kingdom

www.radcliffe-oxford.com
Electronic catalogue and worldwide online ordering facility.

First Edition 1995
Second Edition 1996
Third Edition 1997

British Library Cataloguing in Publication Data.

A catalogue record for this book is available from the British Library.

ISBN-13: 978 185775 734 7

Typeset by Pindar NZ, Auckland, New Zealand.

Printed and bound by Hobbs the Printers, Southampton, UK.

Contents

Foreword

This book is an excellent addition to the knowledge base underlying the delivery of high-quality primary clinical care. It is 10 years since the author, Dr Smith, last pulled together a collection of the most authoritative clinical guidelines in an easily digestible format. At the time, most of the original sources were only available in paper form. Now a whole plethora of information covering primary to tertiary care is available online, and to the busy primary-care clinician this can be overwhelming. This is, therefore, a different book from the previous edition. It is no longer a collection of all available guidelines – there are other encyclopaedic tomes that fulfil that role. Instead, this is unashamedly a selection of the guidelines relevant to primary care that Dr Smith finds most useful in his daily practice as a very experienced general practitioner.

Dr Smith has included various resources that I also have found useful but difficult to locate, even online. He has drawn on a variety of authoritative sources in preparing this collection. In England, a major source of guidance on major clinical topics is the National Institute for Health and Clinical Excellence (NICE). Another source of first-class, accessible clinical decision support is the Scottish Intercollegiate Guidelines Network (SIGN), which, for example, collaborated with the British Thoracic Society to produce the asthma guidelines. A further excellent source that has emerged recently is the online Clinical Knowledge Summaries, the collection previously known as PRODIGY.

The job of the generalist is one of the most demanding in clinical care, and yet it is central to a responsive, effective health service. For that reason alone, I recommend this publication without any reservation at all. I know it will make life easier and more fulfilling for all of us in primary care, and even more importantly, it will ensure that our patients will benefit from care based on the very best of evidence. I suspect non-generalist clinicians will find this book essential reading too. I congratulate the author on a real labour of love, detail and assiduity.

Dr David Colin-Thomé OBE
National Clinical Director for Primary Care
September 2008

Introduction

The world has changed a great deal since I last pulled together a collection of national clinical guidelines. The range of such guidelines has increased exponentially each year, and the evidence to support them has strengthened considerably. A good example of this improvement in knowledge can be seen in the case of diabetes, where we are beginning to understand not only the benefits of treatment but also when to curb our therapeutic zeal, as indicated by the recent results of the ACCORD trial (see diabetic section for details). I have, therefore, once again included my top-10 references, ranging from the seminal (such as the 4S simvastatin study and the ACCORD study) to the interesting (furry pets in eczema, initial consideration of 'new' lamotrigine in 1987). Along with these, there are the patient education diagrams – ones I produce almost daily to illustrate points to my patients. I am particularly pleased to be able to include the children's BMI charts, which I hope will assist us in getting to grips with the increasing problem of childhood obesity.

A healthy change has been the fairly recent move away from 'local guidelines prepared by local clinicians for local people', which always implied that local physiology somehow differed from national norms. The move towards the national assessment of evidence and cost-effectiveness through the National Institute for Health and Clinical Excellence (NICE) and the Scottish Intercollegiate Guidelines Network (SIGN) is welcome. I would also commend the National Centre for Chronic Disease Prevention and Health Promotion (NCCDPHP) in the US, which produces the excellent children's growth and BMI charts included herein. The NCCDPHP has taken the further step of putting these charts into the public domain and encouraging people to download them from the Internet – even to the extent of including instructions on how to insert a user logo.

I am very grateful to the many individuals who have been so helpful in assisting me with obtaining permissions and materials, particularly people at the Department of Medical Illustration in Manchester, Joan Austoker at the National Cancer Screening Programme and colleagues at Clinical Knowledge Summaries, SIGN and NICE, to mention but a few.

I have learnt a huge amount during the collation and preparation of these guidelines. I hope that primary care colleagues in general practice, nursing and pharmacy, as well as registrars, trainees and students, will find them equally useful.

Finally, I'd like to note that these guidelines have been provided in order to assist in your decision-making; they cannot replace sound clinical judgement in the holistic management of individual patients.

Dr Peter Smith
September 2008

About the author

Dr Smith has been a GP in Kingston upon Thames for 19 years. During that time he has been involved in setting up many collaborative ventures, including multifunds and a GP out-of-hours co-operative, Thamesdoc. For several years he was Chairman of the National Association of Primary Care and is now its President. As Chair he was instrumental in the development and implementation of Personal Medical Services (PMS) and practice-based commissioning (PBC).

Peter has a major interest in quality improvement in primary care, which drove him to produce this book. His practice, Churchill Medical Centre, is one of the few recipients of the RCGP Quality Practice Award and has driven innovation in many areas, including extended opening hours, children's services and prescribing quality. He is also Director of Primary Care for United Health Primary Care, developing high-quality general practice in deprived areas, which reflects his interest in tackling health inequalities. In addition, he chairs two NHS Working in Partnership Programmes developing practical systems supporting self-care for patients and for those working in the NHS.

Acknowledgements

This book is dedicated to Linda, Max and Emma, who have patiently tolerated my obsession with producing this collection.

Many of the world's leading clinicians have spent considerable time and effort in producing these guidelines. Every effort has been made to ensure that the necessary permissions have been obtained to use this material and that original authors and publishers have been appropriately credited. I regret any inadvertent omissions and would be happy to include appropriate acknowledgements in future editions.

Every effort has been made to ensure the accuracy of these guidelines, and that the best information available has been used. This does not diminish the requirement to exercise good clinical judgement, and neither the editor nor the original authors can accept any responsibility for their use in practice.

1

ASTHMA

Summary of stepwise management of asthma in adults

Step 3: Add-on therapy

1. Add inhaled long-acting ß2 agonist (LABA)
2. Assess control of asthma:
   Good response to LABA – continue LABA
   Benefit from LABA but control still inadequate – continue LABA and increase inhaled steroid dose to 800mcg/day* (if not already on this dose)
   No response to LABA – stop LABA and increase inhaled steroid to 800mcg/day.* If control still inadequate, institute trial of other therapies, e.g. leukotriene receptor antagonist or SR theophylline

Step 2: Regular preventer therapy

Add inhaled steroid 200–800mcg/day*
400mcg is an appropriate starting dose for many patients
Start at dose of inhaled steroid appropriate to severity of disease

Step 1: Mild intermittent asthma

Inhaled short-acting ß2 agonist as required

*BDP or equivalent

Step 5: Continuous or frequent use of oral steroids

Use daily steroid tablet in lowest dose that provides control
Maintain high-dose inhaled steroid at 2000 mcg/day*
Consider other treatments in order to minimise the use of steroid tablets
Refer patients for specialist care

Step 4: Persistent poor control

Increase inhaled steroid dose up to 2000 mcg/day*
Addition of a fourth drug, e.g. leukotriene receptor antagonist, SR theophylline, ß2 agonist tablet

Patients should start treatment at the step most appropriate to the initial severity of their asthma. Check concordance and reconsider if response to treatment is unexpectedly poor

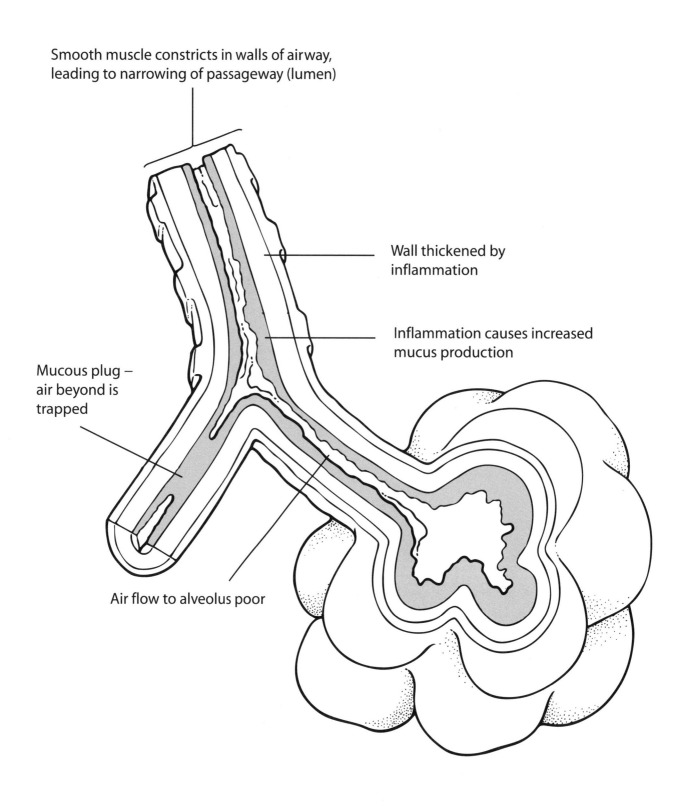

Smooth muscle constricts in walls of airway, leading to narrowing of passageway (lumen)

Wall thickened by inflammation

Inflammation causes increased mucus production

Mucous plug – air beyond is trapped

Air flow to alveolus poor

Figure 1.1 Effects of asthma on airways and alveoli

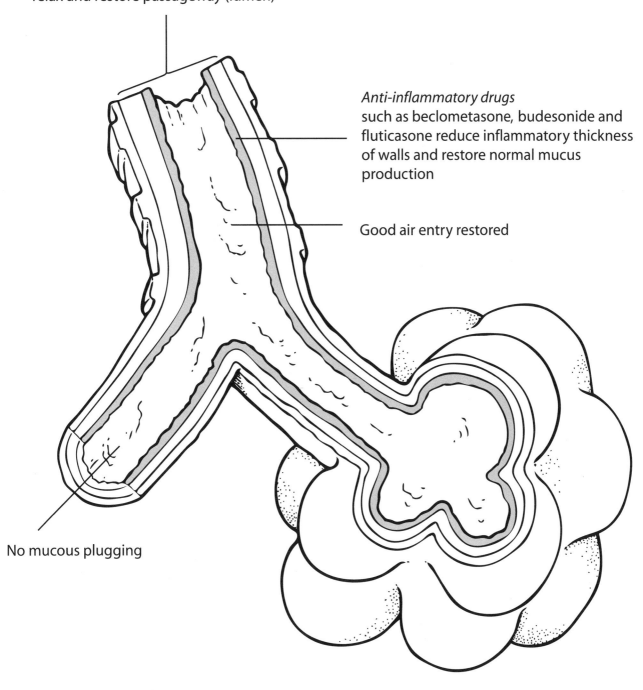

ß agonist drugs
such as salbutamol, terbutaline and
salmeterol cause smooth muscle walls to
relax and restore passageway (lumen)

Anti-inflammatory drugs
such as beclometasone, budesonide and
fluticasone reduce inflammatory thickness
of walls and restore normal mucus
production

Good air entry restored

No mucous plugging

Figure 1.2 Effects of anti-asthmatic drugs

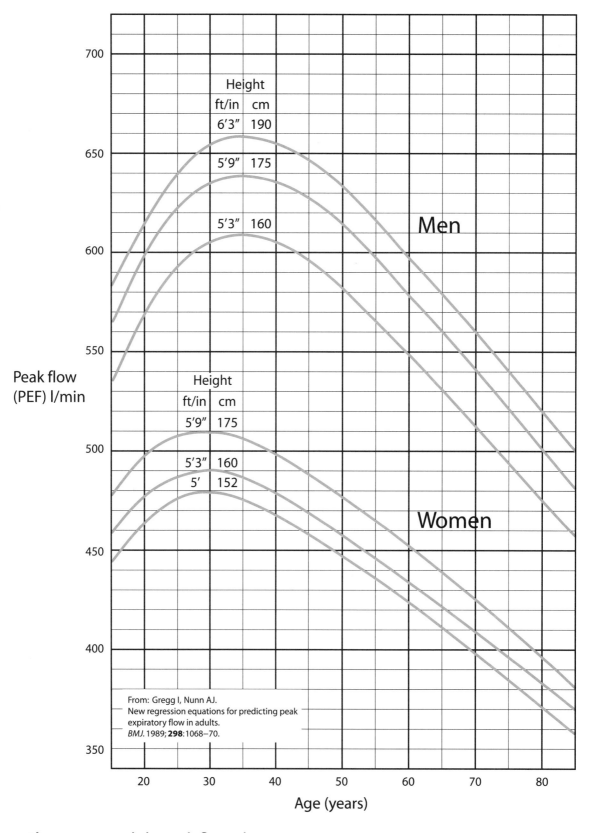

Figure 1.3 Adult peak flow chart

Adult asthma references

This guideline is from the following source:

Scottish Intercollegiate Guidelines Network and British Thoracic Society. *British Guideline on the Management of Asthma: a national clinical guideline*. Edinburgh: SIGN and BTS; 2008. Available at: www.sign.ac.uk/pdf/qrg101.pdf

Ducharme FM. Inhaled glucocorticoids versus leukotriene receptor antagonists as single agent asthma treatment: systematic review of current evidence. *BMJ*. 2003; **326**(7390): 621.

Evidence Based Medicine. High-dose inhaled corticosteroids increase the risk for some systemic adverse effects in asthma. *Evid Based Med*. 1999; **4**(6): 191.

Gallefoss F, Bakke PS. Impact of patient education and self-management on morbidity in asthmatics and patients with chronic obstructive pulmonary disease. *Respir Med*. 2000; **94**(3): 279–87.

Harrison TW, Oborne J, Newton S, *et al*. Doubling the dose of inhaled corticosteroid to prevent asthma exacerbations: randomised controlled trial. *Lancet*. 2004; **363**(9405): 271–5.

Nelson J, Strauss L, Skowronski M, *et al*. Effect of long-term salmeterol treatment on exercise-induced asthma. *N Engl J Med*. 1998; **339**(3): 141–5.

Rodolfo JD, Solarte I, Fitzgerald JM. Asthma. *BMJ Clinical Evidence*. BMJ Publishing Group Ltd. 2005. Available at: www.clinicalevidence.com

Statement by the Royal College of Physicians of London, King's Fund Centre, National Asthma Campaign. Guidelines for management of asthma in adults: I. Chronic persistent asthma [Statement by the British Thoracic Society]. *BMJ*. 1990; **301**: 651–3.

Tee AKH, Koh MS, Gibson PG, *et al*. Long-acting beta2-agonists versus theophylline for maintenance treatment of asthma. *Cochrane Database Syst Rev*. 2007; **2**: CD001281.

Thomson NC, Chaudhuri R, Livingston E. Asthma and cigarette smoking. *Eur Respir J*. 2004; **24**(5): 822–33.

Tierney WM, Rosener JF, Seshadri, R, *et al*. Assessing symptoms and peak expiratory flow rate as predictors of asthma exacerbations. *J Gen Intern Med*. 2004; **19**(3): 237–42.

Summary of stepwise management of asthma in children aged 5–12

Step 3: Add-on therapy

1. Add inhaled long-acting ß2 agonist (LABA)
2. Assess control of asthma:
   Good response to LABA – continue LABA
   Benefit from LABA but control still inadequate – continue LABA and increase
       inhaled steroid dose to 400 mcg/day* (if not already on this dose)
   No response to LABA – stop LABA and increase inhaled steroid to
       400 mcg/day.* If control still inadequate, institute trial of other therapies,
       e.g. leukotriene receptor antagonist or SR theophylline

Step 2: Regular preventer therapy

Add inhaled steroid 200–400 mcg/day*
(or other preventer drug, if inhaled steroid cannot be used)
200 mcg is an appropriate starting dose for many patients
Start at dose of inhaled steroid appropriate to severity of disease

Step 1: Mild intermittent asthma

Inhaled short-acting ß2 agonist as required

*BDP or equivalent

Step 5: Continuous or frequent use of oral steroids

Use daily steroid tablet in lowest dose that provides adequate control
Maintain high-dose inhaled steroid at 800 mcg/day*
Refer to respiratory paediatrician

Step 4: Persistent poor control

Increase inhaled steroid dose up to 800 mcg/day*

Patients should start treatment at the step most appropriate to the initial severity of their asthma. Check concordance and reconsider if response to treatment is unexpectedly poor

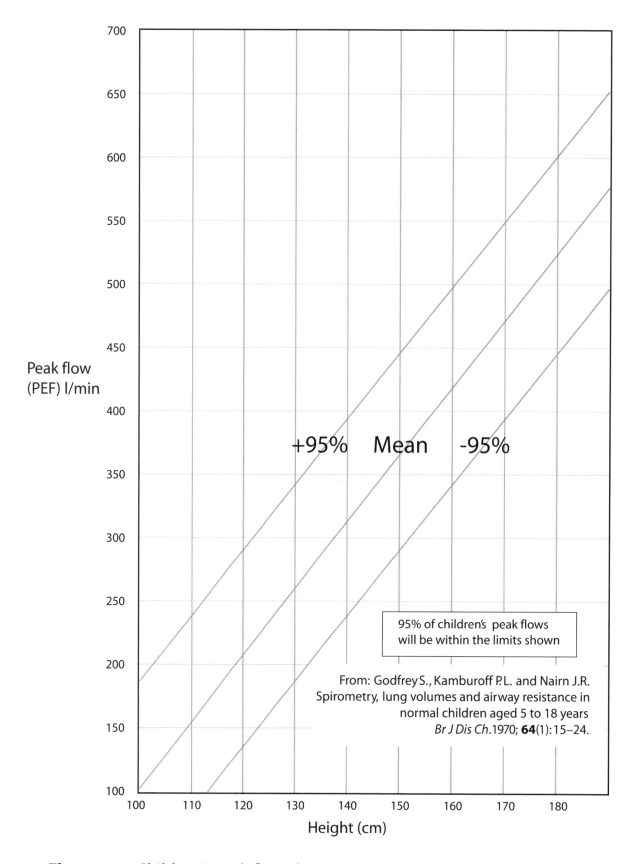

Peak flow (PEF) l/min

Height (cm)

+95%   Mean   -95%

95% of children's peak flows
will be within the limits shown

From: Godfrey S., Kamburoff P.L. and Nairn J.R.
Spirometry, lung volumes and airway resistance in
normal children aged 5 to 18 years
Br J Dis Ch.1970; **64**(1):15–24.

Figure 1.4 Children's peak flow chart

Children's asthma references

This guideline is based upon the following source:

Scottish Intercollegiate Guidelines Network and British Thoracic Society. *British Guideline on the Management of Asthma: a national clinical guideline*. Edinburgh: SIGN and BTS; 2008. Available at: www.sign.ac.uk/pdf/qrg101.pdf

Agertoft L, Pedersen S. Effect of long-term treatment with inhaled budesonide on adult height in children with asthma. *N Engl J Med*. 2000; **343**(15): 1064–9.

Doull IJ. The effect of asthma and its treatment on growth. *Arch Dis Child*. 2004; **89**(1): 60–3.

Guevara JP, Ducharme FM, Keren R, *et al*. Inhaled corticosteroids versus sodium cromoglycate in children and adults with asthma. *Cochrane Database Systs Rev*. 2006; **2**: CD003558.

Guevara JP, Wolf FM, Grum CM, *et al*. Effects of educational interventions for self management of asthma in children and adolescents: systematic review and meta-analysis. *BMJ*. 2003; **326**(7402): 1308–9.

Knorr B, Franchi LM, Bisgaard H, *et al*. Montelukast, a leukotriene receptor antagonist, for the treatment of persistent asthma in children aged 2 to 5 years. *Pediatrics*. 2001; **108**(3): e48.

National Institute for Health and Clinical Excellence. *Guidance on the Use of Inhaler Systems (Devices) in Children under the Age of 5 Years with Chronic Asthma: NICE technology appraisal guidance 10*. London: NICE; 2000. Available at: www.nice.org.uk/guidance/index.jsp?action=article&o=32074

National Institute for Health and Clinical Excellence. *Inhaler Devices for Routine Treatment of Chronic Asthma in Older Children (Aged 5–15 Years): NICE technology appraisal guidance 38*. London: NICE; 2002. Available at: www.nice.org.uk/TA38

Rachelefsky G. Treating exacerbations of asthma in children: the role of systemic corticosteroids. *Pediatrics*. 2003; **112**(2): 382–97.

Robertson CF. Long-term outcome of childhood asthma. *Med J Aust*. 2002; **177**(Suppl): S42–4.

Townshend J, Hails S, McKean M. Diagnosis of asthma in children. *BMJ*. 2007; **335**(7612): 198–202.

2

ATRIAL FIBRILLATION

Atrial fibrillation care pathway

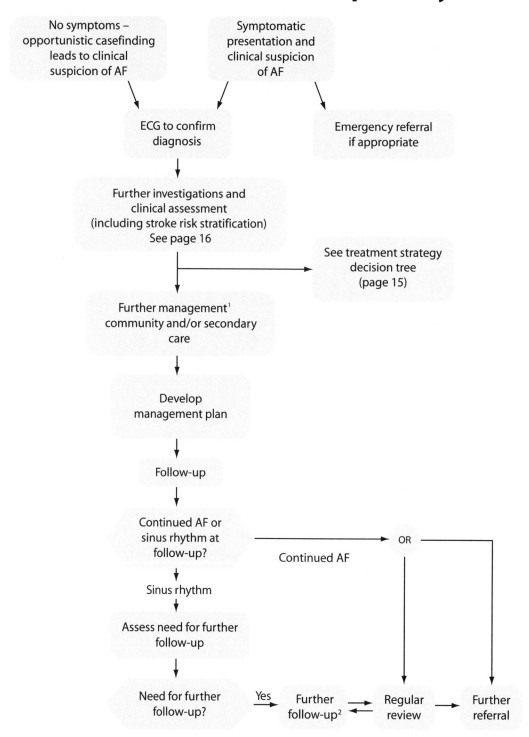

No symptoms – opportunistic casefinding leads to clinical suspicion of AF

Symptomatic presentation and clinical suspicion of AF

ECG to confirm diagnosis

Emergency referral if appropriate

Further investigations and clinical assessment (including stroke risk stratification) See page 16

See treatment strategy decision tree (page 15)

Further management[1] community and/or secondary care

Develop management plan

Follow-up

Continued AF or sinus rhythm at follow-up?

Continued AF

OR

Sinus rhythm

Assess need for further follow-up

Need for further follow-up?

Yes

Further follow-up[2]

Regular review

Further referral

[1] Further management to include rate- or rhythm-control treatment strategy and appropriate antithrombotic therapy based on stroke risk stratification model.
[2] Further follow-up for coexisting conditions and assessment for ongoing anticoagulation.

Atrial fibrillation treatment strategy decision tree

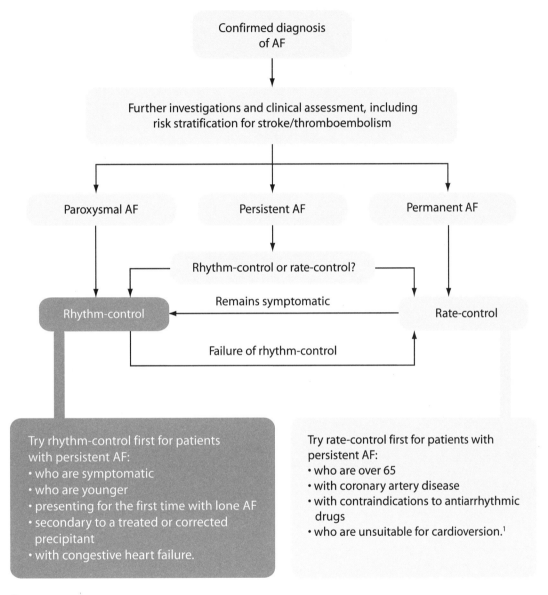

Confirmed diagnosis of AF

Further investigations and clinical assessment, including risk stratification for stroke/thromboembolism

Paroxysmal AF

Persistent AF

Permanent AF

Rhythm-control or rate-control?

Remains symptomatic

Rhythm-control

Rate-control

Failure of rhythm-control

Try rhythm-control first for patients with persistent AF:
• who are symptomatic
• who are younger
• presenting for the first time with lone AF
• secondary to a treated or corrected precipitant
• with congestive heart failure.

Try rate-control first for patients with persistent AF:
• who are over 65
• with coronary artery disease
• with contraindications to antiarrhythmic drugs
• who are unsuitable for cardioversion.[1]

In all cases:
    • explain to the patient the advantages and disadvantages of each strategy before you decide which to use
    • take into account comorbidities when deciding which to use
    • use appropriate antithrombotic therapy.

[1]Patients unsuitable for cardioversion include those with: contraindications to anticoagulation; structural heart disease (e.g. large left atrium >5.5 cm, mitral stenosis) that precludes long-term maintenance of sinus rhythm; a long duration of AF (usually >12 months); a history of multiple failed attempts at cardioversion and/or relapses, even with concomitant use of antiarrhythmic drugs or non-pharmacological approaches; an ongoing but reversible cause of AF (e.g. thyrotoxicosis).

Stroke risk stratification and thromboprophylaxis

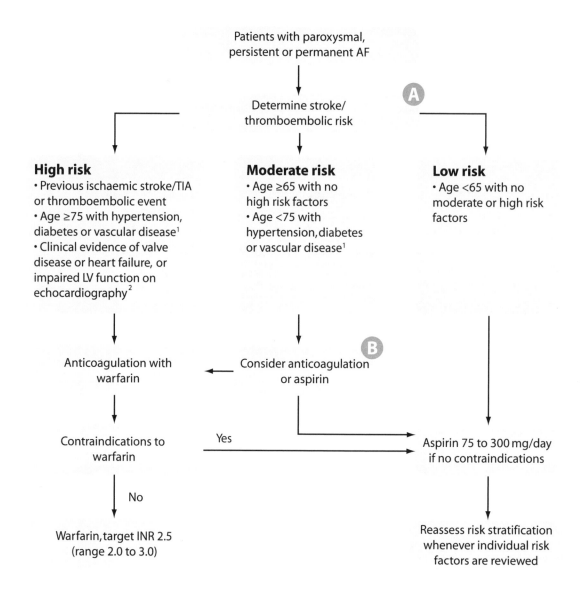

Patients with paroxysmal, persistent or permanent AF
→
Determine stroke/thromboembolic risk

(A)

High risk
• Previous ischaemic stroke/TIA or thromboembolic event
• Age ≥75 with hypertension, diabetes or vascular disease[1]
• Clinical evidence of valve disease or heart failure, or impaired LV function on echocardiography[2]

Moderate risk
• Age ≥65 with no high risk factors
• Age <75 with hypertension, diabetes or vascular disease[1]

Low risk
• Age <65 with no moderate or high risk factors

Anticoagulation with warfarin

Consider anticoagulation or aspirin **(B)**

Contraindications to warfarin

Yes →

Aspirin 75 to 300 mg/day if no contraindications

No ↓

Warfarin, target INR 2.5 (range 2.0 to 3.0)

Reassess risk stratification whenever individual risk factors are reviewed

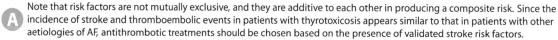

(A) Note that risk factors are not mutually exclusive, and they are additive to each other in producing a composite risk. Since the incidence of stroke and thromboembolic events in patients with thyrotoxicosis appears similar to that in patients with other aetiologies of AF, antithrombotic treatments should be chosen based on the presence of validated stroke risk factors.

(B) Owing to a lack of sufficient clear-cut evidence, treatment may be decided on an individual basis, and the physician must balance the risks and benefits of warfarin versus aspirin. As stroke risk factors are cumulative, warfarin may, for example, be used in the presence of two or more moderate stroke risk factors. Referral and echocardiography may help in cases of uncertainty.

[1] Coronary artery disease or peripheral artery disease.
[2] An echocardiogram is not needed for routine assessment, but it refines clinical risk stratification in the case of moderate or severe LV dysfunction and valve disease.

Atrial fibrillation references

Excerpts from:

National Institute for Health and Clinical Excellence. *The Management of Atrial Fibrillation: NICE guideline 36*. London: NICE; 2006. Available at: www.nice.org. uk/CG36

Reproduced with permission.

Camm AJ, Savelieva I, Lip GY and the Guideline Development Group for the NICE clinical guideline for the management of atrial fibrillation. Rate control in the medical management of atrial fibrillation [review]. *Heart.* 2007; **93**(1): 35–8.

European Atrial Fibrillation Trial Study Group. Secondary prevention in non-rheumatic atrial fibrillation after transient ischaemic attack or minor stroke. *Lancet.* 1993; **342**: 1255–62.

Gheorghiade M, van Veldhuisen DJ, Colucci WS. Contemporary use of digoxin in the management of cardiovascular disorders [review]. *Circulation.* 2006; **113**(21): 2556–64.

Hart RG, Benavente O, McBride R, *et al.* Antithrombotic therapy to prevent stroke in patients with atrial fibrillation: a meta-analysis. *Ann Intern Med.* 1999; **131**: 492–501.

Hart RG, Pearce LA, Aguilar MI. Meta-analysis: antithrombotic therapy to prevent stroke in patients who have nonvalvular atrial fibrillation. *Ann Intern Med.* 2007; **146**(12): 857–67.

Hart RG, Pearce LA, Koudstaal PJ. Transient ischemic attacks in patients with atrial fibrillation: implications for secondary prevention: the European Atrial Fibrillation Trial and Stroke Prevention in Atrial Fibrillation III trial. *Stroke.* 2004; **35**: 948–51.

Lip GY, Tse HF. Management of atrial fibrillation [review]. *Lancet.* 2007; **370**(9587): 604–18.

Stroke Prevention in Atrial Fibrillation Investigators. Lessons from the stroke prevention in atrial fibrillation trials. *Ann Intern Med.* 2003; **138**: 831–8.

Stroke Prevention in Atrial Fibrillation II Investigators. Warfarin versus aspirin for prevention of thromboembolism in atrial fibrillation: *Lancet.* 1994; **343**: 687–91.

Sulke N, Sayers F, Lip GY and the Guideline Development Group for the NICE clinical guideline for the management of atrial fibrillation. Rhythm control and cardioversion. *Heart.* 2007; **93**(1): 29–34.

3

BREAST DISEASE

Referral for breast disease

URGENT REFERRALS

If you suspect that your patient has breast cancer, you should make an urgent referral. GPs are encouraged to do this using same-day direct booking systems such as electronic media, telephone or fax.

It is important that you should only use the classification 'urgent' for those patients whose symptoms are highly suggestive of breast cancer. The main features of this group will be:

- a discrete lump (see below) in the appropriate age group (see below)
- definite signs of cancer, such as:
  ulceration
  skin nodules
  skin distortion.

Other presentations of breast cancer are much less common, e.g. nipple discharge or pain in the absence of a lump.

SUMMARY

Conditions that require referral to a surgeon with a special interest in breast disease:

Lump
- Any new discrete lump.
- New lump in pre-existing nodularity.
- Asymmetrical nodularity that persists at review after menstruation.
- Abscess.
- Cyst persistently refilling or recurrent cyst.

Pain
- Pain associated with a lump.
- Intractable pain not responding to reassurance, to simple measures such as wearing a well-supporting bra, or to common drugs.
- Unilateral persistent pain in post-menopausal women.

Nipple discharge
- Women under 50 with:
  bilateral discharge sufficient to stain clothes
  bloodstained discharge
  persistent single-duct discharge.
- All women aged 50 and over.

Nipple retraction or distortion, nipple eczema

Change in skin contour

Family history
- Request for assessment by a woman with a strong family history of breast cancer.

Breast lump

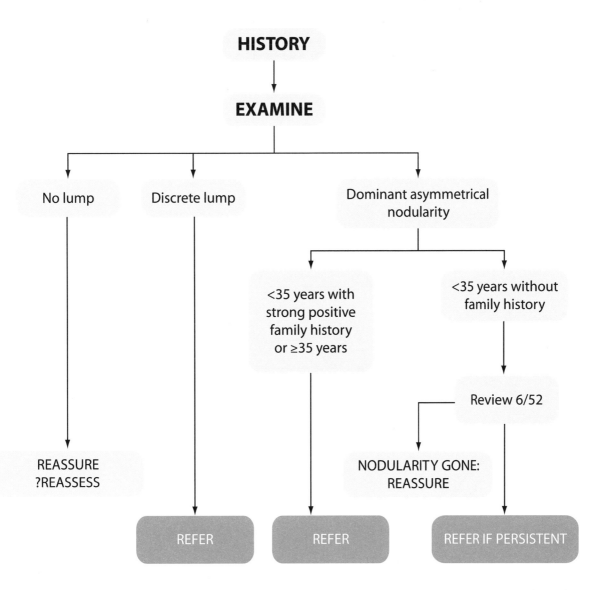

HISTORY

EXAMINE

No lump

Discrete lump

Dominant asymmetrical nodularity

<35 years with strong positive family history or ≥35 years

<35 years without family history

Review 6/52

REASSURE ?REASSESS

NODULARITY GONE: REASSURE

REFER

REFER

REFER IF PERSISTENT

URGENT REFERRALS: see previous page, 'Referral for breast disease'

Nipple discharge

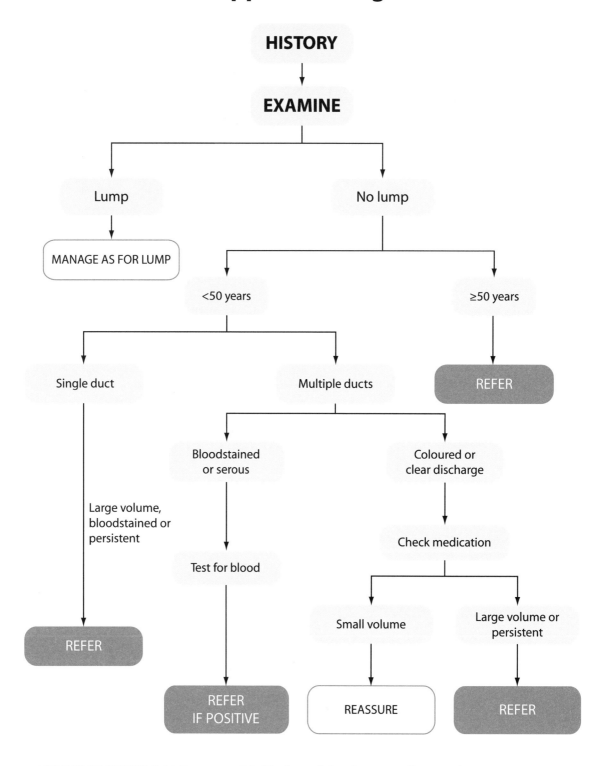

URGENT REFERRALS: see p. 20, 'Referral for breast disease'

Severe cyclical mastalgia

Protocol for treating severe cyclical mastalgia (mild/moderate mastalgia requires examination and reassurance)

The Medicines Control Agency (MCA) – predecessor to the Medicines and Healthcare products Regulatory Agency (MHRA) – made the decision to withdraw the marketing authorisations for products containing gamolenic acid following a review by the Committee on Safety of Medicines (CSM) and the Medicines Commission. The CSM and Medicines Commission came to the conclusion that the data did not support the current standard of effectiveness required for authorisation of these products as medicines for the treatment of breast pain and eczema.

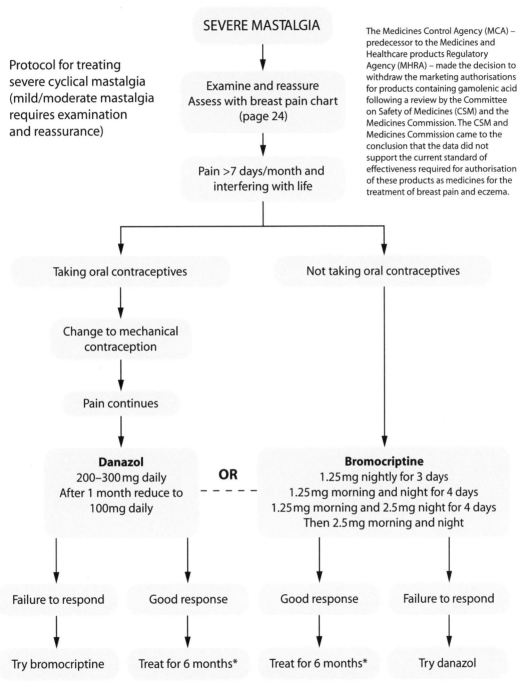

SEVERE MASTALGIA

Examine and reassure
Assess with breast pain chart
(page 24)

Pain >7 days/month and interfering with life

Taking oral contraceptives

Not taking oral contraceptives

Change to mechanical contraception

Pain continues

Danazol
200–300 mg daily
After 1 month reduce to
100 mg daily

OR

Bromocriptine
1.25 mg nightly for 3 days
1.25 mg morning and night for 4 days
1.25 mg morning and 2.5 mg night for 4 days
Then 2.5 mg morning and night

Failure to respond

Good response

Good response

Failure to respond

Try bromocriptine

Treat for 6 months*

Treat for 6 months*

Try danazol

* After 6 months, treatment should be stopped. Breast pain will recur in only half of patients, and some of these will not need further treatment because pain is milder.
Severe recurrences can be treated with a further course of previously successful treatment.

Breast pain

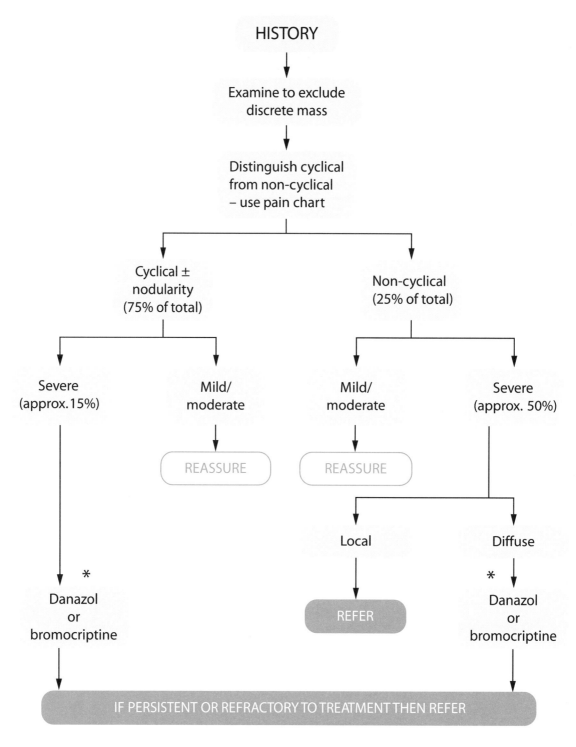

HISTORY

↓

Examine to exclude
discrete mass

↓

Distinguish cyclical
from non-cyclical
– use pain chart

**Cyclical ±
nodularity
(75% of total)**

**Non-cyclical
(25% of total)**

Severe
(approx.15%)

Mild/
moderate

Mild/
moderate

Severe
(approx. 50%)

REASSURE

REASSURE

Local

Diffuse

*

Danazol
or
bromocriptine

REFER

*

Danazol
or
bromocriptine

IF PERSISTENT OR REFRACTORY TO TREATMENT THEN REFER

* Local management protocols
may differ. Please discuss
with your local breast unit.

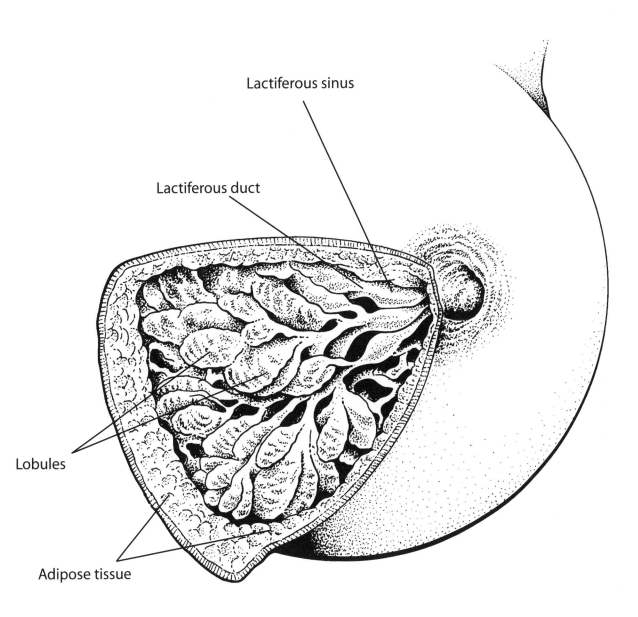

Lactiferous sinus

Lactiferous duct

Lobules

Adipose tissue

Figure 3.1 The breast during lactation

Breast references

These breast guidelines are from a masterpiece of clarity:

Austoker J, Mansel R, Baum M, *et al. Guidelines for Referral of Patients with Breast Problems*. 2nd edn. Sheffield: NHS Cancer Screening Programmes; 2004.

Australian National Breast Cancer Centre. *The investigation of a new breast symptom – a guide for GPs*. New South Wales: National Breast Cancer Centre; 2006. Available at: www.nbcc.org.au/bestpractice/resources/IBS172_theinvestigationofan.pdf

Barclay M, Carter D, Horobin JM, *et al.* Patterns of presentation of breast disease over ten years in a specialised clinic. *Health Bull.* 1991; **49**: 229–36.

Duijm LE, Guit GL, Hendriks JH, *et al.* Value of breast imaging in women with painful breasts: observational follow up study. *BMJ.* 1998; **317**(7171): 1492–5.

Khan SA, Apkarian AV. The characteristics of cyclical and non-cyclical mastalgia: a prospective study using a modified McGill Pain Questionnaire. *Breast Cancer Res Treat.* 2002; **75**(2): 147–57.

Matherne TH, Green A Jr, Tucker JA, *et al.* Fibromatosis: the breast cancer imitator [review]. *South Med J.* 2004; **97**(11): 1100–3.

Mehta TS. Current uses of ultrasound in the evaluation of the breast [review]. *Radiol Clin North Am.* 2003; **41**(4): 841–56.

Nosarti C, Crayford T, Roberts JV, *et al.* Delay in presentation of symptomatic referrals to a breast clinic: patient and system factors. *Br J Cancer.* 2000; **82**(3): 742–8.

Pharoah PDP, Day NE, Duffy S, *et al.* Family history and the risk of breast cancer: a systematic review and meta-analysis. *Int J Cancer.* 1997; **71**: 800–9.

Roberts MM, Elton RA, Robinson SE, *et al.* Consultations for breast disease in general practice and hospital referral patterns. *Br J Surg.* 1987; **74**: 1020–2.

Santen RJ, Mansel R. Benign breast disorders [review]. *N Engl J Med.* 2005; **353**(3): 275–85.

4

CERVICAL CYTOLOGY

Cervical cytology results 1

Result: Negative

Explanation	Action
No nuclear abnormalities identified	Ensure the patient is informed of the result The term 'normal' should be used to inform the woman of her screening result Recall as and if appropriate – see below

Recall

Patient's history	Recall interval
No previous cervical screening history	Routine recall
Previous screening results negative	Routine recall
Aged 65* and over with no previous negative screening history	Three negative tests, 3 years apart, then no further recall
Previous abnormal screening	For minor abnormalities (borderline and mild dyskaryosis) follow protocol for the particular abnormality See below
Previously treated for CIN	Follow up protocol for patients treated for CIN See below
Previous CIN1 (not treated)	At least 3 negative tests, 6–12 months apart, then routine recall

*Over 60 years in Scotland

Result: Inadequate

Explanation	Action
About 9% of all conventional smears are inadequate Insufficient or unsuitable material present Inadequate fixation of smears Poor spreading of smears Smear consisted mainly of blood and pus or inflammatory exudate Excessive cytolysis may render samples unsuitable	Repeat sample immediately after treating any infection or atrophy, preferably within 3 months Repeat sample as soon as convenient if technically inadequate If persistent (3 inadequate samples), advise assessment by colposcopy. The rate of inadequate results may reduce if liquid based cytology (LBC) is introduced.

Cervical cytology results 2

Result: Negative but with incidental findings

Explanation

No nuclear abnormalities present

Incidental observations include vaginal infections without evidence of dyskaryosis or borderline nuclear change

Action

Investigate and manage infection as appropriate

Ensure patient is informed of the result whilst being aware of the social consequences of a diagnosis of a sexually transmitted disease. The woman may not be aware that this result may be reported as a consequence of cervical screening

If asymptomatic, the woman may not be expecting a report of a possible infection

Recall if and as appropriate for a negative result

Result: Borderline nuclear abnormality

Explanation

Approximately 5% of all samples show borderline nuclear change or mild dyskaryosis

Nuclear changes that cannot be described as normal

Samples in which there is doubt as to whether or not the nuclear changes reflect true dyskaryosis

Borderline nuclear change is most often reported in the presence of HPV-type changes

From this:
• The majority of women with borderline results will have ensuing samples that revert to normal

• Those who do not should be managed appropriately (see action) and are highly unlikely to develop cervical cancer

Action

Repeat sample within 6 months for changes bordering on mild dyskaryosis, particularly in association with HPV. The majority of smears will return to normal by this stage. If there is an associated treatable condition, treat and repeat screen at no more than 6 months

If changes persist (3 borderline results) refer for colposcopy

Three consecutive negative results, 6 months apart, required before returning to routine recall

Repeat sample in 3–6 months when the differential diagnosis is between benign/reactive changes and higher degrees of dyskaryosis or ?glandular neoplasia. The laboratory may recommend a repeat screening in a shorter interval, or that gynaecological referral should be considered

If in a 10-year period there are 3 borderline or more severe results, refer to colposcopy

Cervical cytology results 3

Result: Mild dyskaryosis

Explanation

Approximately 5% of all samples show borderline nuclear change or mild dyskaryosis

Nuclear abnormalities reflecting probable CIN1 (i.e. low grade CIN). Mild dyskaryosis is often associated with HPV

From this:
- The majority of women with mild dyskaryosis will have ensuing results that revert to normal
- Those who do not should be managed appropriately (see action) and are highly unlikely to develop cervical cancer

Action

- Repeat sample in 6 months. Many will have returned to normal by this stage
- Refer for colposcopy if changes persist on 2 occasions If a single mild dyskaryotic result is obtained after treatment for CIN2 or worse, refer for colposcopy
- Three consecutive negative results, 6 months apart, required before returning to routine recall
- If in a 10-year period there are 3 borderline or more severe results, refer for colposcopy

Result: Moderate dyskaryosis

Explanation

Approximately 1% of all samples show moderate dyskaryosis

Nuclear abnormalities reflecting probable presence of CIN2, which should be managed as suspected high-grade CIN

Action

Refer for colposcopy

Result: Severe dyskaryosis

Explanation

Approximately 0.5% of all samples show severe dyskaryosis

Nuclear abnormalities reflecting probable presence of CIN3 (high grade CIN)

Action

Refer for colposcopy

Result: Severe dyskaryosis ?invasive carcinoma

Explanation

Less than 0.1% of samples suggest invasive carcinoma

Nuclear and cellular abnormalities indicating probable CIN3 with additional features suggesting possibility of invasive cancer

Action

Urgent referral to a gynaecological oncologist

Result: Glandular neoplasia or ?glandular neoplasia

Explanation

Dyskaryotic glandular cells. May represent:
- endocervical adenocarcinoma *in situ* or
- endocervical adenocarcinoma of the cervix or
- adenocarcinoma of the endometrium or
- extra-uterine adenocarcinomas

Action

Urgent referral to a gynaecological oncologist

Note: Adenocarcinoma *in situ* may coexist with CIN3, and it may not always be possible to distinguish them cytologically.

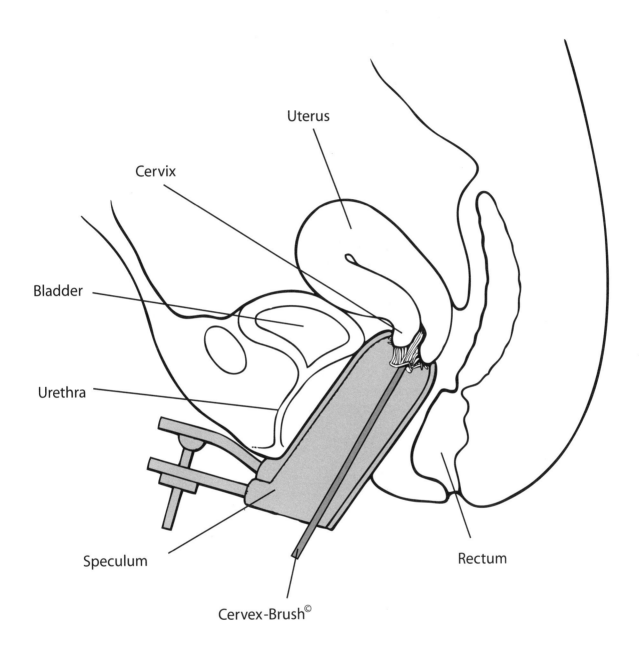

Figure 4.1 Diagram of smear being taken using Cervex-Brush©

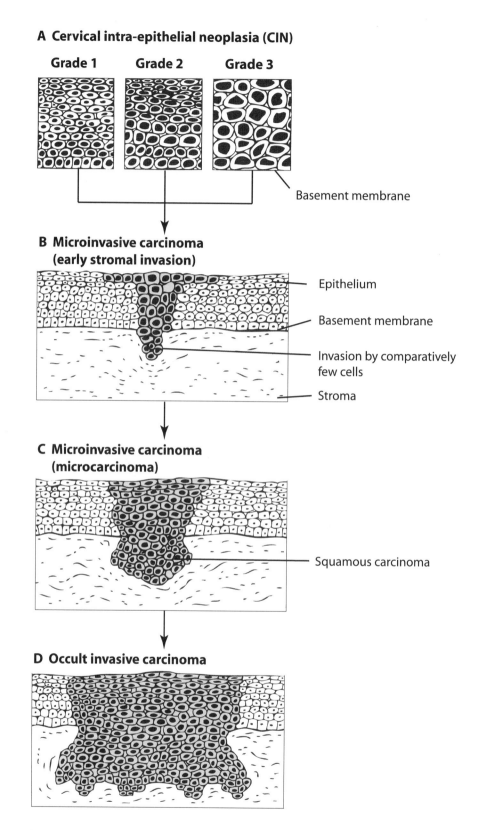

A Cervical intra-epithelial neoplasia (CIN)

Grade 1   Grade 2   Grade 3

Basement membrane

B Microinvasive carcinoma (early stromal invasion)

Epithelium

Basement membrane

Invasion by comparatively few cells

Stroma

C Microinvasive carcinoma (microcarcinoma)

Squamous carcinoma

D Occult invasive carcinoma

Figure 4.2 Development of carcinoma from CIN

Cervical cytology references

These cytology guidelines are an excerpt from:

National Health Service Cervical Screening Programme. *Cervical Screening Results Explained: A Guide for Primary Care.* 2nd edn. Sheffield: NHSCSP Publications; 2003.

Arbyn M, Bergeron C, Klinkhamer P, *et al.* Liquid compared with conventional cervical cytology: a systematic review and meta-analysis [review]. *Obstet Gynecol.* 2008; **111**(1): 167–77.

Austoker J. Cancer prevention in primary care: screening for cervical cancer. *BMJ.* 1994; **309**(6949): 241–8.

Dey P, Collins S, Desai M, *et al.* (1996) Adequacy of cervical cytology sampling with the Cervex brush and the Aylesbury spatula: a population based randomised controlled trial. *BMJ.* **313**(7059): 721–3. Erratum in: *BMJ.* 1996; **313**(7063): 978.

National Coordinating Network (National Cervical Screening Programme), British Society for Clinical Cytology, Royal College of Pathologists' Working Party. Borderline nuclear changes in cervical smears: guidelines on their recognition and management. *J Clin Pathol.* 1994; **47**: 481–92.

National Health Service Cervical Screening Programme. *Guidelines for Clinical Practice and Programme Management.* 2nd edn. Sheffield: NHSCSP Publications; 1997.

National Institute for Health and Clinical Excellence. *Cervical Cancer–Cervical Screening (Review): NICE technology appraisal guidance 69.* London: NICE; 2003. Available at: www.nice.org.uk/nicemedia/pdf/TA69_LBC_review_A4summary.pdf

Pichichero ME. Who should get the HPV vaccine? [review]. *J Fam Pract.* 2007; **56**(3): 197–202.

Schiffman M, Castle PE, Jeronimo J, *et al.* Human papillomavirus and cervical cancer [review]. *Lancet.* 2007; 370(9590): 890–907.

Williamson SL, Hair T, Wadehra V. The effects of different sampling techniques on smear quality and the diagnosis of cytological abnormalities in cervical screening. *Cytopathology.* 1997; **8**(3): 188–95.

Wright TC Jr, Massad LS, Dunton CJ, *et al.* American Society for Colposcopy and Cervical Pathology-sponsored Consensus Conference. 2006 consensus guidelines for the management of women with abnormal cervical cancer screening tests [review]. *Am J Obstet Gynecol.* 2007; **2197**(4): 346–55.

5

COPD

Stable chronic obstructive pulmonary disease

Patients with COPD should have access to the wide range of skills available from a multidisciplinary te

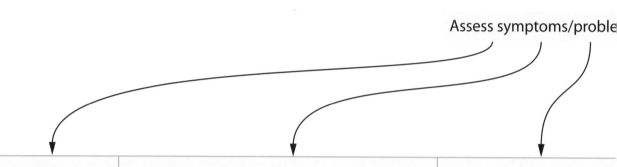

Assess symptoms/proble

Smoking	Breathlessness and exercise limitation	Frequent exacerbations
• Offer help to stop smoking at every opportunity. • Combine pharmacotherapy with appropriate support as part of a programme.	*(Stop therapy if ineffective)* Use short-acting bronchodilator as needed (ß2-agonist or anticholinergic). If still symptomatic, try combined therapy with a short-acting ß2-agonist and a short-acting anticholinergic. If still symptomatic, use a long-acting bronchodilator (ß2-agonist or anticholinergic). In moderate or severe COPD: if still symptomatic, consider a combination of a long-acting bronchodilator and inhaled corticosteroid; discontinue if no benefit after 4 weeks. If still symptomatic, consider adding theophylline.	• Offer annual influenza vaccination. • Offer pneumococcal vaccination. • Give self-management advice.
	Offer pulmonary rehabilitation to all patients who consider themselves functionally disabled (usually MRC grade 3 and above). Consider referral for surgery: bullectomy, lung volume reduction, transplantation.	Optimise bronchodilator therapy with one or more long-acting bronchodilator (ß2-agonist or anticholinergic). Add inhaled corticosteroids if FEV1 ≤50% and two or more exacerbations in a 12-month period (NB: these will usually be used with long-acting bronchodilators).

Palliative care
• Opiates can be used for the palliation of breathlessness in patie
with end-stage COPD unresponsive to other medical therapy.

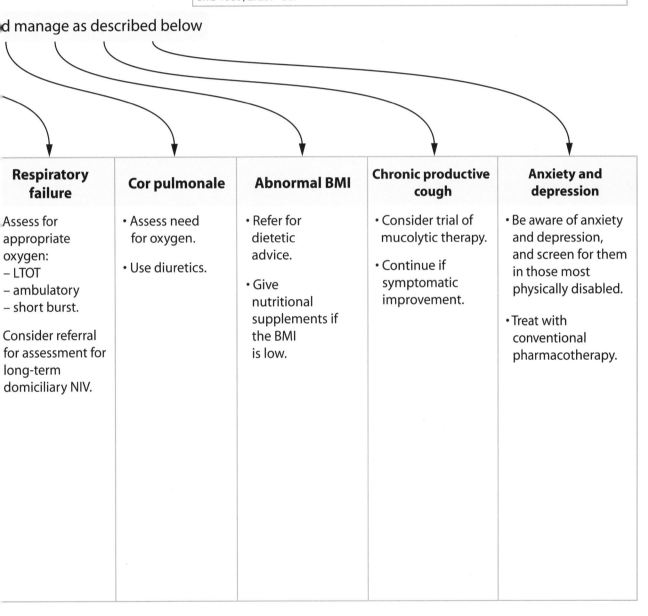

ith COPD

d manage as described below

Respiratory failure	Cor pulmonale	Abnormal BMI	Chronic productive cough	Anxiety and depression
Assess for appropriate oxygen: – LTOT – ambulatory – short burst. Consider referral for assessment for long-term domiciliary NIV.	• Assess need for oxygen. • Use diuretics.	• Refer for dietetic advice. • Give nutritional supplements if the BMI is low.	• Consider trial of mucolytic therapy. • Continue if symptomatic improvement.	• Be aware of anxiety and depression, and screen for them in those most physically disabled. • Treat with conventional pharmacotherapy.

Use benzodiazepines, tricyclic antidepressants, major tranquillisers and oxygen when appropriate.
nvolve multidisciplinary palliative care teams.

Diagnosing COPD

Definition of COPD
COPD is characterised by airflow obstruction. The airflow obstruction is usually progressive,
is not fully reversible and does not change markedly over several months.
The disease is predominantly caused by smoking.

Consider the diagnosis of COPD for patients who are:
• over 35
• smokers or ex-smokers
• have any of these symptoms:
   – exertional breathlessness
   – chronic cough
   – regular sputum production
   – frequent winter 'bronchitis'
   – wheeze
• and have no clinical features of asthma (see table below).

↓

Perform spirometry if COPD seems likely.
Airflow obstruction is defined as:
• FEV1 <80% predicted
• and FEV1/FVC <0.7.
Spirometric reversibility testing is not usually necessary as part of the diagnostic process or to plan initial therapy.

↓

If still in doubt about diagnosis, consider the following pointers:
• clinically significant COPD is not present if FEV1 and FEV1/FVC ratio return to normal with drug therapy
• asthma may be present if:
   – there is a >400ml response to bronchodilators
   – serial peak flow measurements show significant diurnal or
     day-to-day variability
   – there is a >400ml response to 30mg prednisolone daily for 2 weeks
• refer for more detailed investigations if needed.

↓   ↓

If still in doubt, make a provisional diagnosis and start empirical treatment   If no doubt, diagnose COPD and start treatment

↓   ↓

Reassess diagnosis in view of response to treatment

Clinical features differentiating COPD and asthma		
	COPD	**Asthma**
Smoker or ex-smoker	Nearly all	Possibly
Symptoms under age 35	Rare	Common
Chronic productive cough	Common	Uncommon
Breathlessness	Persistent and progressive	Variable
Night-time waking with breathlessness and/or wheeze	Uncommon	Common
Significant diurnal or day-to-day variability of symptoms	Uncommon	Common

COPD references

These algorithms are from the very comprehensive NICE guideline:
National Institute for Health and Clinical Excellence. *Management of Chronic Obstructive Pulmonary Disease in Adults in Primary and Secondary Care: NICE guideline 1.* London: NICE; 2005. Available at: www.nice.org.uk/CG1
Reproduced with permission.

Lipworth BJ. Systemic adverse effects of inhaled corticosteroid therapy: a systematic review and meta-analysis. *Arch Intern Med.* 1999; **159**(9): 941–55.

National Collaborating Centre for Chronic Conditions. *Chronic Obstructive Pulmonary Disease: national clinical guideline on management of chronic obstructive pulmonary disease in adults in primary and secondary care.* London: Royal College of Physicians of London; 2004. Available at: www.thorax.bmj.com/content/vol59/suppl_1/

O'Neill B, Mahon JM, Bradley J. Short-burst oxygen therapy in chronic obstructive pulmonary disease. *Respir Med.* 2006; **100**(7): 1129–38.

Ram FS. Use of theophylline in chronic obstructive pulmonary disease: examining the evidence. *Curr Opin Pulm Med.* 2006; **12**(2): 132–9.

Royal Pharmaceutical Society of Great Britain. *Practice Guidance on the Care of People with Asthma and Chronic Pulmonary Disease.* London: RPSGB; 2006.

Salpeter SR, Buckley NS, Salpeter EE. Meta-analysis: anticholinergics, but not beta-agonists, reduce severe exacerbations and respiratory mortality in COPD. *J Gen Intern Med.* 2006; **21**(10): 1011–19.

Scottish Intercollegiate Guidelines Network. *Community Management of Lower Respiratory Tract Infection in Adults.* Edinburgh: SIGN; 2002. Available at: www.sign.ac.uk/guidelines/fulltext/59/index.html

Silverman EK, Speizer FE. Risk factors for the development of chronic obstructive pulmonary disease. *Med Clin North Am.* 1996; **80**(3): 501–22.

Sin DD, Wu L, Anderson JA, *et al.* Inhaled corticosteroids and mortality in chronic obstructive pulmonary disease. *Thorax.* 2005; **60**(12): 992–7.

Vincken W, van Noord JA, Greefhorst AP, *et al.* Improved health outcomes in patients with COPD during 1 year's treatment with tiotropium. *Eur Respir J.* 2002; **19**(2): 209–16.

6

CORONARY
HEART DISEASE

Risk factor assessment charts for primary prevention of cardiovascular disease

Notes on the use of the charts

The Joint British Societies guidelines for the prevention of cardiovascular disease in clinical practice' indicated that the use of these charts is not appropriate for people who have existing atherosclerotic disease or are at higher risk for other medical reasons.
The following are examples of patients for whom these charts are not appropriate:
- those with CHD or other major atherosclerotic disease
- those with familial hypercholesterolaemia or other inherited dyslipidaemias
- those with renal dysfunction including diabetic nephropathy
- those with type 1 and 2 diabetes mellitus.

CVD risk is also higher than indicated in the charts for:
- those with a family history of premature CVD or stroke (male first-degree relatives aged >55 years and female first-degree relatives aged <65 years), which increases the risk by a factor of approximately 1.3
- those with raised triglyceride values (>1.7 mmol/l)
- women with premature menopause
- those who are not yet diabetic, but have impaired fasting glycaemia or impaired glucose tolerance.

In some ethnic minorities the risk charts underestimate CVD risk, because they have not been validated in these populations. For example, in people originating from the Indian subcontinent it is safest to assume that the CVD risk is higher than predicted from the charts (1.4 times).

The guidelines also stated that these charts are based on groups of people with untreated blood pressure, total cholesterol and HDL cholesterol values. In people already receiving antihypertensive therapy for whom a decision is to be made about whether to introduce lipid-lowering medication, or vice versa, the charts can only act as a guide. Unless recent pre-treatment risk factor values are available, it is generally safest to assume that CVD risk is higher than that predicted by current levels of blood pressure or lipids on treatment.

To estimate an individual's total 10-year risk of developing CVD, choose the table for his or her sex, lifetime smoking status, and age. Within this square define the level of risk according to the point where the coordinates for systolic blood pressure and the ratio of total cholesterol to high density lipoprotein (HDL) cholesterol meet. If no HDL cholesterol result is available, then assume this is 1.0mmol/l and the lipid scale can be used for total cholesterol alone.

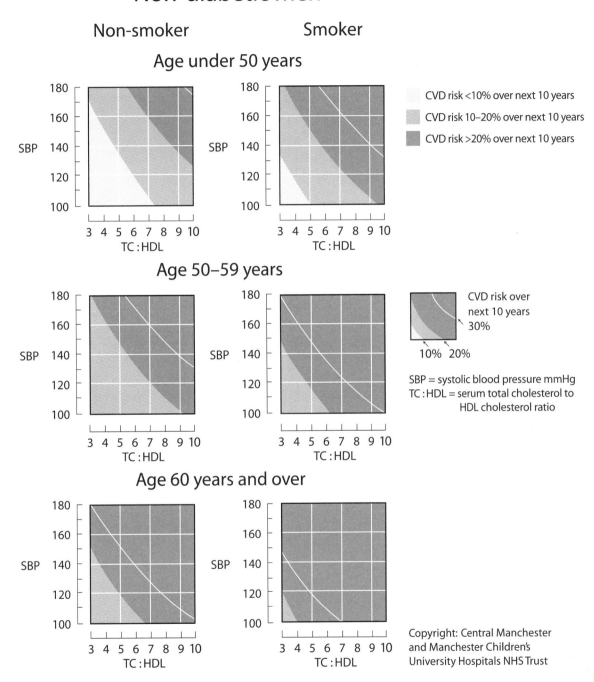

Figure 6.1 Risk factor assessment for primary prevention of cardiovascular disease – non-diabetic men

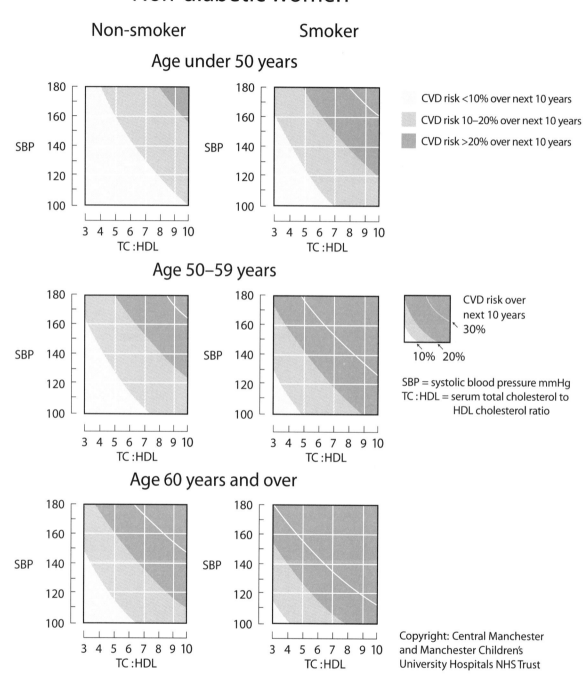

Figure 6.2 Risk factor assessment for primary prevention of cardiovascular disease – non-diabetic women

Lipid modification:
assessment of CVD risk in primary care
for primary prevention

Identifying people for full formal risk assessment

If the person has a history of CHD, angina, stroke or TIA, peripheral vascular disease, diabetes or a monogenic lipid disorder, do not include in risk assessment process, as these patients are already considered at high risk

Is person 75 or over?

YES → Consider at increased risk of CVD, and likely to benefit from statin treatment, particularly if person smokes or has high blood pressure. Consider comorbidities, benefits and risks of treatment, and person's preference

NO

Use systematic strategy rather than opportunistic assessment to identify people aged 40–74 who are likely to be at high risk

Estimate risk using risk factors already recorded in primary care electronic medical records

10-YEAR RISK LESS THAN 20%

10-YEAR RISK 20% OR GREATER

Prioritise for full formal risk assessment
Arrange discussion of risk assessment

Review risk on an ongoing basis

Discuss process of risk assessment, including option to decline assessment

RISK ASSESSMENT DECLINED

Communication about risk assessment and treatment

Encourage the person to work with you to reduce their CVD risk.

- Find out what they have been told about their risk and how they feel about it.
- Explore their beliefs about what determines future health.

- Assess their readiness to change lifestyle, undergo tests and take medication.
- Tell them about possible future management options.
- Develop a shared management plan.
- Check that they have understood what has been discussed.

Inform people that risk is estimated, but is more likely to be accurate if over 20%.

Offer people information about their absolute risk of CVD and treatment (including benefits and harms) over a 10-year period. The information should:
- present individualised risk and benefit scenarios
- present the absolute risk of events numerically
- use appropriate diagrams and text.

Lipid modification:
full formal risk assessment

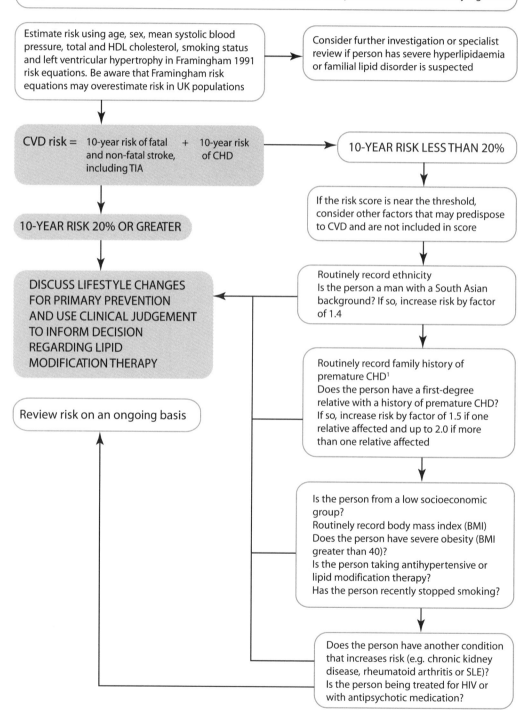

Healthcare professionals should always be aware that all CVD risk estimation tools can provide only an approximation of CVD risk. Interpretation of CVD risk scores should always reflect informed clinical judgement.

Estimate risk using age, sex, mean systolic blood pressure, total and HDL cholesterol, smoking status and left ventricular hypertrophy in Framingham 1991 risk equations. Be aware that Framingham risk equations may overestimate risk in UK populations

Consider further investigation or specialist review if person has severe hyperlipidaemia or familial lipid disorder is suspected

CVD risk = 10-year risk of fatal and non-fatal stroke, including TIA + 10-year risk of CHD

10-YEAR RISK LESS THAN 20%

10-YEAR RISK 20% OR GREATER

If the risk score is near the threshold, consider other factors that may predispose to CVD and are not included in score

Routinely record ethnicity
Is the person a man with a South Asian background? If so, increase risk by factor of 1.4

DISCUSS LIFESTYLE CHANGES FOR PRIMARY PREVENTION AND USE CLINICAL JUDGEMENT TO INFORM DECISION REGARDING LIPID MODIFICATION THERAPY

Routinely record family history of premature CHD[1]
Does the person have a first-degree relative with a history of premature CHD? If so, increase risk by factor of 1.5 if one relative affected and up to 2.0 if more than one relative affected

Review risk on an ongoing basis

Is the person from a low socioeconomic group?
Routinely record body mass index (BMI)
Does the person have severe obesity (BMI greater than 40)?
Is the person taking antihypertensive or lipid modification therapy?
Has the person recently stopped smoking?

Does the person have another condition that increases risk (e.g. chronic kidney disease, rheumatoid arthritis or SLE)?
Is the person being treated for HIV or with antipsychotic medication?

[1] Age at onset younger than 55 in fathers, sons or brothers or younger than 65 in mothers, daughters or sisters.

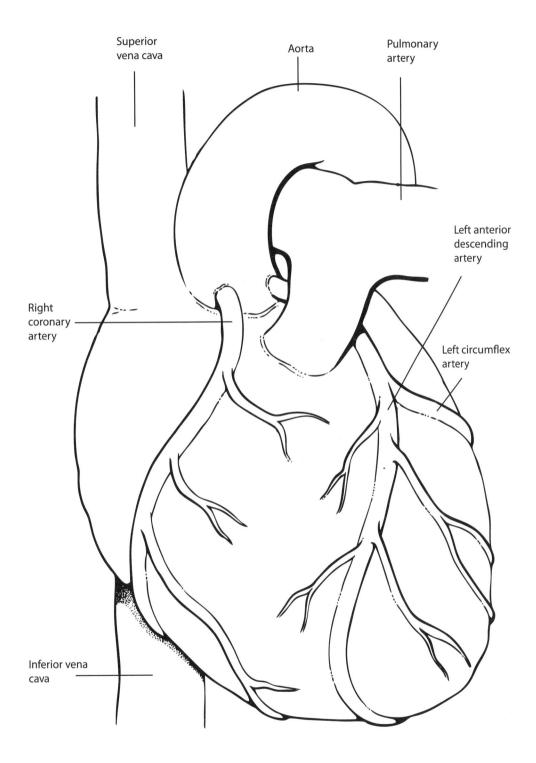

Superior
vena cava

Aorta

Pulmonary
artery

Left anterior
descending
artery

Right
coronary
artery

Left circumflex
artery

Inferior vena
cava

Figure 6.3 Main coronary arteries

Lipid modification therapy

Primary prevention

Consider drugs for primary and secondary prevention for morbidi*

Offer 40 mg simvastatin (or drug of similar efficacy and acquisition cost) as part of the management strategy for adults over 40 who have a 20% or greater 10-year risk of developing CVD, based on Framingham 1991 10-year risk equations and clinical judgement

If there are potential drug interactions or 40 mg simvastatin is contraindicated, offer a lower dose of simvastatin or pravastatin

Do not routinely offer:
• higher intensity statins
• fibrates
• anion exchange resins.

Do not offer nicotinic acid or the combination of an anion exchange resin, fibrate or a fish oil supplement with a statin

There is no target level for total or LDL cholesterol for primary prevention

Review drug therapy in line with good clinical practice

Repeat lipid profile is not necessary but review management according to clinical judgement and patient preference

Ongo

Measure liver function within 3 months and at 12 months, but not again unless clinically indicated

If drugs that interfere with statin metabolism are introduced for another illness, consider reducing the statin dose or stopping it temporarily or permanently

Advise people to seek medical advice if they develop muscle pain, tenderness or weakness

If statins are not tolerated for primary prevention, consider:
• fibrates   • anion exchange resins   • ezetimibe[1]

[1] See National Institute for Health and Clinical Excellence. *Ezetimibe for the Treatment of Primary (heterozygous-familial and non-familial) Hypercholesterolaemia: NICE technology appraisal 132.* London: NICE; 2005.

Lipid modification therapy

...is evidence in clinical trials of beneficial effect on CVD ...lity outcomes

Offer lipid modification therapy as soon as possible

Offer 40 mg simvastatin (or drug of similar efficacy and acquisition cost) to all adults with clinical evidence of CVD

If there are potential drug interactions or 40 mg simvastatin is contraindicated, offer a lower dose of simvastatin or pravastatin

Offer a higher intensity statin to people with acute coronary syndrome. Do not delay until lipid levels are available. Take into account:
• informed preference
• other drug therapy
• comorbidities
• benefits and risks.

Consider increasing dose to 80 mg simvastatin or drug of similar efficacy and cost if the total cholesterol does not fall below 4 mmol/l or the LDL cholesterol does not fall below 2 mmol/l. Take into account:

• informed preference
• comorbidities
• other drug therapy
• benefits and risks.

Use an 'audit' level of total cholesterol of 5 mmol/l to assess progress in groups with CVD. Recognise that less than half of patients will achieve total cholesterol less than 4 mmol/l or LDL cholesterol less than 2 mmol/l

Measure fasting lipid levels about 3 months after the start of treatment

...nitoring

Do not routinely monitor creatine kinase in people without adverse events, but do measure it in people with muscle symptoms

Stop statins and seek specialist advice if unexplained peripheral neuropathy develops

If statins are not tolerated for secondary prevention, consider:
• fibrates
• anion exchange resins
• nicotinic acid
• ezetimibe[1]

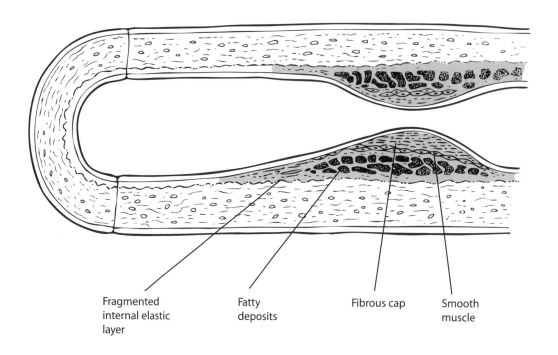

Fragmented
internal elastic
layer

Fatty
deposits

Fibrous cap

Smooth
muscle

Figure 6.4 Atheromatous plaque

Primary prevention CHD references

These are the excellent charts used in the extremely authoritative Joint British Societies' guidelines. They were prepared by Professor Paul Durrington and are copyright of Central Manchester and Manchester Children's University Hospital NHS Trust Department of Medical Illustration, whose staff were very helpful in providing the original artwork.

Joint British Societies. JBS 2: Joint British Societies' guidelines on prevention of cardiovascular disease in clinical practice. *Heart.* 2005; **91**(Suppl. 5): S1–52.

Brindle PM, McConnachie A, Upton MN, *et al.* The accuracy of the Framingham risk-score in different socioeconomic groups: a prospective study. *Br J Gen Pract.* 2005; **55**(520): 838–45.

Colhoun HM, Betteridge DJ, Durrington PN, and the CARDS investigators. Primary prevention of cardiovascular disease with atorvastatin in type 2 diabetes in the Collaborative Atorvastatin Diabetes Study (CARDS): multicentre randomised placebo-controlled trial. *Lancet.* 2004; **364**: 685–96.

Collins R, Armitage J, Parish S, *et al.* Heart Protection Study Collaborative Group MRC/BHF Heart Protection Study of cholesterol-lowering with simvastatin in 5,963 people with diabetes: a randomised placebo-controlled trial. *Lancet.* 2003; **361**: 2005–16.

Department of Health. *National Policy on Statin Prescribing.* London: DH; 2006. Available at: www.heart.nhs.uk/CHD/28050/28154/Statins%20-%20 National%20Policy%20Statement%207%2011%2006.doc

Department of Health. *National Service Framework for Coronary Heart Disease.* London: DH; 2000. Available at: www.dh.gov.uk/en/Publicationsandstatistics/ Publications/PublicationsPolicyAndGuidance/DH_4094275

Royal Pharmaceutical Society of Great Britain. *Practice guidance on sale of over-the-counter statins.* London: RPSGP; 2004. Available at: www.rpsgb.org.uk/pdfs/ otcsimvastatinguid.pdf

Scandinavian Simvastatin Survival Study Group. Randomised trial of cholesterol lowering in 4,444 patients with coronary heart disease: the Scandinavian Simvastatin Survival Study (4S). *Lancet.* 1994; **344**: 1383–9.

Shepherd J, Cobbe SM, Ford I and the West of Scotland Coronary Prevention Study Group (WOSCOPS). Prevention of coronary heart disease with pravastatin in men with hypercholesterolaemia. *New Engl J Med.* 1995; **333**: 1301–7.

Thavendiranathan P, Bagai A, Brookhart MA, *et al.* Primary prevention of cardiovascular diseases with statin therapy: a meta-analysis of randomized controlled trials [review]. *Arch Intern Med.* 2006; **166**(21): 2307–13.

Tunstall-Pedoe H, Woodward M. By neglecting deprivation, cardiovascular risk scoring will exacerbate social gradients in disease. *Heart.* 2006; **92**(3): 307–10.

Lipid modification guideline reference

The lipid modification guideline was produced by NICE as we were going to press. For appropriate references please see the sections on angina, secondary prevention of MI and primary prevention of CHD.

National Institute for Health and Clinical Excellence. *Lipid Modification: cardiovascular risk assessment and the modification of blood lipids for the primary and secondary prevention of cardiovascular disease: NICE guideline 67*. London: NICE; 2008. Available at: www.nice.org.uk/CG67

Reproduced with permission.

Stable angina

Clinical assessment

Some patients describe discomfort and heaviness or breathlessness, rather than pain. Chest discomfort, irrespective of site, is more likely to be angina when precipitated by exertion and relieved by rest. It is also characteristically relieved by glyceryl trinitrate.

Characteristic features of stable angina include:

- tight, dull or heavy feeling of discomfort
- discomfort often retrosternal or left side of chest and can radiate to left arm, neck, jaw and back
- often brought on with exertion or emotional stress and eased with rest
- symptoms typically last up to several minutes after exertion or emotional stress has stopped
- other factors – may be precipitated by cold weather or following a meal.

Suspected angina – initial assessment

Detailed initial clinical assessment including:

- history
- examination
- BP
- hb
- TFT
- cholesterol.
- glucose

Early referral to secondary care

- New-onset angina.
- Established CHD with increase in symptoms.

Diagnosis

Initial investigation

Should usually be investigated by:
- baseline electrocardiogram and
- exercise tolerance test.

C

If unable to undergo ETT or has pre-existing ECG abnormalities, should be considered for myocardial perfusion scintigraphy

B

Further investigation

Coronary angiography should be considered after non-invasive testing where patients are:
- identified to be at high risk or
- diagnosis remains unclear.

Following initial assessment in primary care, patients with suspected angina should, wherever possible, have the diagnosis confirmed and the severity of the underlying coronary heart disease assessed in the chest pain evaluation service that offers the earliest appointment, regardless of model.

D

Key: **A B C D** Indicates grade of recommendation ☑ Good practice point

Management of stable angina

Pharmacological management

FIRST-LINE THERAPY

A ß blockers should be used as first-line therapy for the relief of symptoms of stable angina

→

A Patients who are intolerant of ß blockers should be treated with either rate-limiting calcium channel blockers, long-acting nitrates or nicorandil

NITRATES

A Sublingual glyceryl trinitrate tablets or spray should be used for the immediate relief of angina and before performing activities that are known to bring on angina

COMBINATION THERAPY

A When adequate control of anginal symptoms is not achieved with beta-blockade, a calcium channel blocker should be added

→

☑ Rate-limiting calcium channel blockers should be used with caution when combined with ß blockers

☑ Patients whose symptoms are not controlled on maximum therapeutic doses of two drugs should be considered for referral to a cardiologist

DRUG INTERVENTIONS TO PREVENT NEW VASCULAR EVENTS

A All patients with stable angina due to atherosclerotic disease should receive long-term standard aspirin and statin therapy

A All patients with stable angina should be considered for treatment with angiotensin-converting enzyme inhibitors

Revascularisation

ALL PATIENTS

☑ Coronary artery bypass grafting and percutaneous coronary interventions are both appropriate options for the alleviation of anginal symptoms

PATIENTS WITH TRIPLE VESSEL DISEASE

A Patients with triple vessel disease should be considered for coronary artery bypass grafting to improve prognosis, but where unsuitable they should be offered percutaneous coronary intervention

PATIENTS WITH LEFT MAIN STEM DISEASE

A Patients with significant left main stem disease should undergo coronary artery bypass grafting

PATIENTS WITH SINGLE/DOUBLE VESSEL DISEASE

A Patients with single or double vessel disease, where optimal medical therapy fails to control angina symptoms, should be offered percutaneous coronary intervention, or where unsuitable, they should be considered for coronary artery bypass grafting

Key: **A B C D** Indicates grade of recommendation | ☑ Good practice point

Angina references

Scottish Intercollegiate Guidelines Network. (2007) *Management of Stable Angina: SIGN guideline 96.* Edinburgh: SIGN; 2007. Available at: www.sign.ac.uk/pdf/qrgchd.pdf

Berger JS, Brown DL, Becker RC. Low-dose aspirin in patients with stable cardiovascular disease: a meta-analysis [review]. *Am J Med.* 2008; **121**(1): 43–9.

Bravata DM, Gienger AL, McDonald KM, *et al.* Systematic review: the comparative effectiveness of percutaneous coronary interventions and coronary artery bypass graft surgery [review]. *Ann Intern Med.* 2007; **147**(10): 703–16.

Department of Health. *National service framework for coronary heart disease.* London: DH; 2000. Available at: www.dh.gov.uk/en/Publicationsandstatistics/Publications/PublicationsPolicyAndGuidance/DH

Fox K, Garcia MA, Ardissino D, *et al.* Guidelines on the management of stable angina pectoris: executive summary. *Eur Heart J.* 2006; **27**(11): 1341–81.

Jacobson TA. Secondary prevention of coronary artery disease with omega-3 fatty acids [review]. *Am J Cardiol.* 2006; **98**(4A): 61–70i.

Kumar S, Hall RJ. Drug treatment of stable angina pectoris in the elderly: defining the place of calcium channel antagonists. *Drugs Aging.* 2003; **20**(11): 805–15.

Lopez-Sendon J, Swedberg K, McMurray J, *et al.* Expert consensus document on beta-adrenergic receptor blockers. *Eur Heart J.* 2004; **25**(15): 1341–62.

Metz LD, Beattie M, Hom R, *et al.* The prognostic value of normal exercise myocardial perfusion imaging and exercise echocardiography: a meta-analysis [review]. *J Am Coll Cardiol.* 2007; **49**(2): 227–37.

Scirica BM, Morrow DA. Troponins in acute coronary syndromes [review]. *Prog Cardiovasc Dis.* 2004; **47**(3): 177–88.

Tunstall-Pedoe H, Woodward M, Tavendale R, *et al.* Comparison of the prediction by 27 different factors of coronary heart disease and death in men and women of the Scottish Heart Health Study: cohort study. *BMJ.* 1997; **315**(7110): 722–9.

Drug therapy – after an MI in the last 12 months 1

Offer all patients who have had an acute MI treatment with a combination of the following drugs:
• ACE inhibitor
• aspirin
• beta blocker
• statin.

ACE inhibitors

• Offer ACE inhibitors early after presentation and titrate upwards to the maximum tolerated or target dose.
• Do not routinely prescribe ARBs unless the patient is intolerant or allergic to an ACE inhibitor.
• Continue ACE inhibitors indefinitely in patients with preserved LV function or LVSD, whether or not they have heart failure symptoms.
• Early after an acute MI, do not routinely use the combination of ACE inhibitor/ARB for patients with heart failure and/or LVSD.
Assessment/monitoring
• Assess LV function in all patients who have had an MI.
• Measure renal function, serum electrolytes and BP before starting an ACE inhibitor or ARB and again within 1 or 2 weeks.
• Monitor patients as the dose is titrated and more frequently for patients at increased risk of deterioration in renal function.
• Monitor patients with chronic heart failure in line with *NICE clinical guideline 5*.

Antiplatelet therapy

• Offer aspirin and continue indefinitely.
• Do not offer clopidogrel alone as first-line therapy, but consider it for patients with aspirin hypersensitivity.
• If the patient has not been treated with a combination of aspirin and clopidogrel during the acute phase of an MI, do not routinely initiate this combination.
• The combination of aspirin and clopidogrel is not recommended for any longer than 12 months after the acute phase of MI, unless there are other indications to continue dual antiplatelet therapy. The combination is usually recommended for a shorter duration after a STEMI.
• Clopidogrel in combination with low-dose aspirin is recommended in the management of non-ST-segment-elevation acute coronary syndrome in people who are at moderate to high risk of MI or death. It is recommended that this combination is continued for 12 months after the most recent acute episode. Thereafter standard care, including low-dose aspirin alone, is recommended.[1] For patients after a STEMI treated with the combination of aspirin and clopidogrel during the first 24 hours, this combination should be continued for at least 4 weeks. Thereafter standard treatment, including low-dose aspirin, should be given unless there are other indications to continue dual antiplatelet therapy.
• For patients with a history of dyspepsia, consider a PPI and low-dose aspirin. Refer to *NICE clinical guideline 17*.
• For patients with a history of aspirin-induced ulcer bleeding whose ulcers have healed and who are H. pylori negative, consider a full-dose PPI and low-dose aspirin. Refer to *NICE clinical guideline 17*.
Assessment/monitoring
• The risk of MI or death in patients presenting with non-ST-segment-elevation acute coronary syndrome can be determined by clinical signs and symptoms, plus one or both of the following:
– clinical investigations indicating ongoing myocardial ischaemia
– raised blood levels of markers of cardiac cell damage, such as troponin.[1]

Beta blockers

• Offer a beta blocker as soon as the patient is clinically stable and titrate upwards to the maximum tolerated dose. Continue treatment indefinitely.
• For patients with LVSD being offered treatment, a beta blocker licensed for use in heart failure may be preferred.

Potassium channel activators

• Nicorandil is not recommended to reduce cardiovascular risk.

[1] This recommendation is from *Clopidogrel in the Treatment of Non-ST-Segment-Elevation Acute Coronary Syndrome: NICE technology appraisal guidance 80*. It has been incorporated into this guideline in line with NICE procedures for developing clinical guidelines.

Drug therapy – after an MI in the last 12 months 2

Vitamin K antagonists

- High-intensity warfarin (INR >3) should not be considered as an alternative to aspirin in first-line treatment.
- For patients unable to take aspirin or clopidogrel, consider moderate-intensity warfarin (INR 2–3) for up to 4 years and possibly longer.
- For patients unable to take clopidogrel and at low risk of bleeding, consider treatment with aspirin and moderate-intensity warfarin (INR 2–3) combined.
- The combination of warfarin and clopidogrel is not routinely recommended.
- Continue warfarin for patients already being treated for another indication. Consider adding aspirin for patients being treated with moderate-intensity warfarin (INR 2–3) who are at low risk of bleeding.

Calcium channel blockers

- Do not routinely use calcium channel blockers for secondary prevention.
- If beta blockers are contraindicated or need to be discontinued, consider diltiazem or verapamil for secondary prevention in patients without pulmonary congestion or LVSD.[2]
- For patients who are stable, calcium channel blockers may be used to treat hypertension and/or angina. For patients with heart failure, use amlodipine and avoid verapamil, diltiazem and short-acting dihydropyridine agents, in line with *NICE clinical guideline 5*.

Aldosterone antagonists

- For patients with symptoms and/or signs of heart failure and LVSD, initiate treatment with an aldosterone antagonist licensed for post-MI treatment within 3–14 days of the MI, preferably after ACE inhibitor therapy.
- For patients with clinical heart failure and LVSD already being treated with an aldosterone antagonist for a concomitant condition, continue with the aldosterone antagonist or an alternative that is licensed for early post-MI treatment.

Assessment/monitoring
- Monitor renal function and serum potassium before and during treatment. If hyperkalaemia is a problem, halve the dose or stop the treatment.

Statins and other lipid lowering agents

- Statin treatment is recommended for adults with clinical evidence of CVD, and it should be offered as soon as possible.

Refer to *NICE clinical guideline 67* (May 2008). See summary on pages 48-49.
- Discuss the risks and benefits of treatment with the patient, taking into account comorbidities and life expectancy.
- Start therapy with a drug with a low acquisition cost (taking into account required daily dose and product price per dose).
- For patients intolerant of statins, other lipid lowering agents should be considered.
- Reduce or stop the dose of statins if there are issues surrounding the metabolic pathway, food and/or drug interactions and/or concomitant illness.
- Discontinue the statins and seek specialist advice if patients develop peripheral neuropathy that may be attributable to the statin treatment.

Assessment/monitoring
- Measure baseline liver enzymes before initiation.
- Do not routinely exclude patients from treatment who have raised liver enzymes.
- Routine monitoring of creatine kinase in asymptomatic patients is not recommended, but should be measured in patients who develop muscle symptoms.

[2] At the time of initial publication of these guidelines (May 2007), diltiazem and verapamil did not have UK marketing authorisation for this indication. Please refer to the BNF or the most recent data sheet. If unlicensed, informed consent should be obtained and documented.

Drug therapy – after a proven MI in the past (more than 12 months ago) 1

ACE inhibitors

- For patients without heart failure and with preserved LV function, offer an ACE inhibitor and titrate upwards to the maximum tolerated effective dose.
- For patients with LVSD (asymptomatic), offer ACE inhibitor treatment and titrate upwards to the effective clinical dose for patients with heart failure and LVSD.
- For patients with heart failure and LVSD, ACE inhibitor and ARB treatment should be in line with *NICE clinical guideline 5*.
- Continue indefinitely in patients with preserved LV function or LVSD, whether or not they have symptoms of heart failure.
- For patients with LVSD (asymptomatic) who are intolerant or allergic to an ACE inhibitor, substitute an ARB.

Assessment/monitoring
- Assess LV function in all patients who have had an MI.
- Measure renal function, serum electrolytes and BP before starting an ACE inhibitor or ARB, and again within 1 or 2 weeks.
- Monitor patients as the dose is titrated, and more frequently if patients are at increased risk of deterioration in renal function.
- Monitor patients with chronic heart failure in line with *NICE clinical guideline 5*.

Antiplatelet therapy

- Offer aspirin and continue indefinitely.
- Do not offer clopidogrel alone as first-line therapy, but consider it for patients with aspirin hypersensitivity.
- The combination of aspirin and clopidogrel is not recommended for routine use for any longer than 12 months after the acute phase of MI, unless there are other indications to continue dual antiplatelet therapy. The combination is usually recommended for a shorter duration after a STEMI.
- For patients with a history of dyspepsia, consider treatment with a PPI and low-dose aspirin. Refer to *NICE clinical guideline 17*.
- For patients with a history of aspirin-induced ulcer bleeding whose ulcers have healed and who are H. pylori negative, consider a full-dose PPI and low-dose aspirin. Refer to *NICE clinical guideline 17*.

Beta blockers

- Offer treatment with a beta blocker to all patients with LVSD, whether or not they have symptoms.
- Manage patients with heart failure plus LVSD in line with *NICE clinical guideline 5*.
- Do not routinely offer treatment with a beta blocker for patients with preserved LV function who are asymptomatic, unless they are at increased risk of further cardiovascular events, or there are other compelling indications for beta blocker treatment.

Potassium channel activators

- Nicorandil is not recommended to reduce cardiovascular risk.

Drug therapy – after a proven MI in the past (more than 12 months ago) 2

Vitamin K antagonists

- High-intensity warfarin (INR >3) should not be considered as an alternative to aspirin in first-line treatment.
- The combination of warfarin and clopidogrel is not routinely recommended.
- Continue warfarin for patients already being treated for another indication.

Calcium channel blockers

- Calcium channel blockers should not routinely be used for secondary prevention.
- For patients who are stable, calcium channel blockers may be used to treat hypertension and/or angina. For patients with heart failure, use amlodipine and avoid verapamil, diltiazem and short-acting dihydropyridine agents, in line with *NICE clinical guideline 5*.

Aldosterone antagonists

- For patients with heart failure due to LVSD, aldosterone antagonist treatment should be in line with *NICE clinical guideline 5*.

Assessment/monitoring
- Monitor renal function and serum potassium before and during treatment. If hyperkalaemia is a problem, halve the dose or stop the treatment.

Statins and other lipid lowering agents

- Statin treatment is recommended for adults with clinical evidence of CVD and should be offered as soon as possible.

Refer to *NICE guideline 67* (May 2008). Summary on pages 48-49.
- Discuss the risks and benefits of treatment with the patient, taking into account comorbidities and life expectancy.
- Start therapy with a drug with a low acquisition cost (taking into account required daily dose and product price per dose).
- For patients intolerant of statins, consider other lipid lowering agents.
- Reduce or stop the dose of statins if there are issues surrounding the metabolic pathway, food and/or drug interactions and/or concomitant illness.
- Discontinue the statin and seek specialist advice if patients develop peripheral neuropathy that may be attributable to the statin treatment.

Assessment/monitoring
- Measure baseline liver enzymes before initiation.
- Do not routinely exclude patients who have raised liver enzymes from treatment.
- Routine monitoring of creatine kinase in asymptomatic patients is not recommended, but should be measured in patients who develop muscle symptoms.

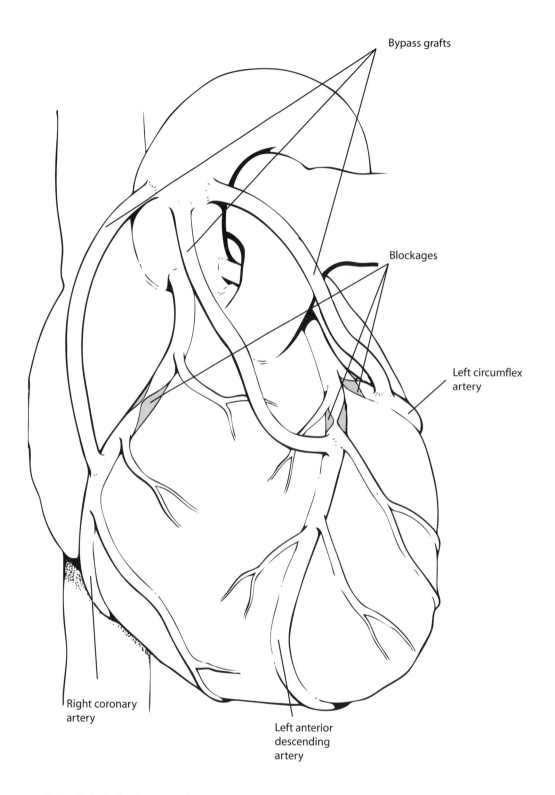

Bypass grafts

Blockages

Left circumflex artery

Right coronary artery

Left anterior descending artery

Figure 6.5 A 'triple bypass'

MI – secondary prevention references

This guideline is an extract from the Quick Reference Guide to:

National Institute for Health and Clinical Excellence. *MI Secondary Prevention: secondary prevention in primary and secondary care for patients following a myocardial infarction: NICE guideline 48*. London: NICE; 2006. Available at: www.nice.org. uk/CG48

Reproduced with permission.

Clark AM, Hartling L, Vandermeer B, *et al*. Meta-analysis: secondary prevention programs for patients with coronary artery disease. *Ann Intern Med*. 2005; **143**(9): 659–72.

Department of Health. *National Policy on Statin Prescribing*. London: DH; 2006. Available at: www.heart.nhs.uk/CHD/28050/28154/Statins%20-%20 National%20Policy%20Statement%207%2011%2006.doc

Fox KM. Efficacy of perindopril in reduction of cardiovascular events among patients with stable coronary artery disease: randomised, double-blind, placebo-controlled, multicentre trial (the EUROPA study). *Lancet*. 2003; **362**(9386): 782–8.

Freemantle N, Cleland J, Young P, *et al*. Beta-blockade after myocardial infarction: systematic review and meta regression analysis. *BMJ*. 1999; **318**(7200): 1730–7.

GISSI-Prevenzione Investigators. Dietary supplementation with n-3 polyunsaturated fatty acids and vitamin E after myocardial infarction: results of the GISSI-Prevenzione trial. *Lancet*. 1999; **354**(9177): 447–55.

Impact of Nicorandil in Angina Study Group. Effect of nicorandil on coronary events in patients with stable angina: the impact of nicorandil in angina (IONA) randomised trial. *Lancet*. 2002; **359**(9314): 1269–75.

Joint British Societies. JBS 2: Joint British Societies' guidelines on prevention of cardiovascular disease in clinical practice. *Heart*. 2005; **91**(Suppl. 5): S1–52.

National Institute for Health and Clinical Excellence. *Clopidogrel in the Treatment of Non-ST-Segment-Elevation Acute Coronary Syndrome: NICE technology appraisal 80*. London: NICE; 2004. Available at: www.nice.org.uk/nicemedia/pdf/ TA080quickrefguide.pdf

The Task Force on Beta-Blockers of the European Society of Cardiology. Expert Consensus Document on Beta-Adrenergic Receptor Blockers. *European Heart Journal*. 2004; **25**(15): 1341–62.

Trichopoulou A, Bamia C, Norat T, *et al*. Modified Mediterranean diet and survival after myocardial infarction: the EPIC-Elderly Study. *Eur J Epidemiol*. 2007; **22**(12): 871–81.

7

DEPRESSION

Depression 1

Step 1: Recognition of depression in primary care and general hospital settings

Screening

- In primary care and general hospital settings, screen patients with:
  - a past history of depression
  - significant physical illnesses causing disability
  - other mental health problems, such as dementia.
- Bear in mind the potential physical causes of depression and the possibility that depression can be caused by medication.

Screening questions

- Use two screening questions, such as:
  - 'During the last month, have you often been bothered by feeling down, depressed or hopeless?' and
  - 'During the last month, have you often been bothered by having little interest or pleasure in doing things?'

Step 2: Treatment of mild depression in primary care

Watchful waiting

- In mild depression, if the patient does not want treatment or may recover with no intervention, arrange further assessment – normally within 2 weeks.

Exercise

- Advise patients of all ages with mild depression of the benefits of following a structured and supervised exercise programme. Effective duration of such programmes is up to 3 sessions per week of moderate duration (45 minutes to 1 hour) for between 10 and 12 weeks.

Guided self-help

- For patients with mild depression, consider a guided self-help programme that consists of the provision of appropriate written materials and limited support over 6 to 9 weeks, including follow up from a professional who typically introduces the self-help programme and reviews progress and outcome.

Computerised cognitive behavioural therapy

- Computerised CBT should be considered for the treatment of mild depression.

Review in mild depression

- Consider contacting all patients with mild depression who do not attend follow-up appointments.

Sleep and anxiety management

- Consider advice on sleep hygiene and anxiety management.

Psychological interventions

- In mild and moderate depression, consider psychological treatment specifically focused on depression (problem-solving therapy, brief CBT and counselling) of 6 to 8 sessions over 10 to 12 weeks.
- Offer the same range of treatments to older people and to younger people.
- In psychological interventions, therapist competence and therapeutic alliance have significant bearing on the outcome of intervention.
- Where significant comorbidity exists, consider extending treatment duration or focusing specifically on comorbid problems.

Antidepressants

- Antidepressants are not recommended for the initial treatment of mild depression, because the risk–benefit ratio is poor.
- Where mild depression persists after other interventions, or is associated with psychosocial and medical problems, consider use of an antidepressant.
- If a patient with a history of moderate or severe depression presents with mild depression, consider use of an antidepressant (see Step 3).

Step 3: Treatment of moderate to severe depression in primary care

Starting treatment

- In moderate depression, offer antidepressant medication to all patients routinely, before psychological interventions.
- Discuss patients' fears of addiction or other concerns about medication. For example, explain that craving and tolerance do not occur.
- When starting treatment, tell patients about:
  - the risk of discontinuation/withdrawal symptoms
  - potential side effects.
- Inform patients about the delay in onset of effect, the time course of treatment and the need to take medication as prescribed. Make available written information appropriate to the patient's needs.

Monitoring risk

- See patients who are considered to be at increased risk of suicide or who are younger than 30 years old 1 week after starting treatment. Monitor frequently until the risk is no longer significant.
- If there is a high risk of suicide, prescribe a limited quantity of antidepressants.
- If there is a high risk of suicide, consider additional support such as more frequent contacts with primary care staff or telephone contacts.
- Monitor for signs of akathisia, suicidal ideas, and increased anxiety and agitation, particularly in the early stages of treatment with an SSRI.
- Advise patients of the risk of these symptoms, and that they should seek help promptly if these are at all distressing.
- If a patient develops marked and/or prolonged akathisia or agitation while taking an antidepressant, review the use of the drug.

Continuing treatment

- See patients who are not considered to be at increased risk of suicide 2 weeks after starting treatment and regularly thereafter
  - for example, every 2–4 weeks in the first 3 months – reducing the frequency if response is good.
- For patients with a moderate or severe depressive episode, continue antidepressants for at least 6 months after remission.
- Once a patient has taken antidepressants for 6 months after remission, review the need for continued antidepressant treatment. This review may include consideration of the number of previous episodes, presence of residual symptoms, and concurrent psychosocial difficulties.

Depression 2

Step 3: Treatment of moderate to severe depression in primary care (cont.)

Choice of antidepressants
- For routine care, use an SSRI, because they are as effective as tricyclic antidepressants and less likely to be discontinued because of side effects.
- Consider using a generic form of SSRI. Fluoxetine or citalopram, for example, would be reasonable choices, because they are generally associated with fewer discontinuation/withdrawal symptoms. Note the higher propensity of fluoxetine for drug interactions.
- Treatments such as dosulepin, phenelzine, combined antidepressants, and lithium augmentation of antidepressants should be routinely initiated only by specialist mental healthcare professionals (including General Practitioners with a Special Interest in Mental Health).
- Consider toxicity in overdose in patients at significant risk of suicide. Note that the highest risk is with tricyclic antidepressants (with the exception of lofepramine), but that venlafaxine is also more dangerous than other equally effective drugs recommended for routine use in primary care.
- Be aware of clinically significant interactions with concomitant drugs (particularly when prescribing fluoxetine, fluvoxamine, paroxetine, tricyclic antidepressants or venlafaxine). Consider consulting appendix 1 of the British National Formulary.
- If increased agitation develops early in treatment with an SSRI, provide appropriate information and, if the patient prefers, either change to a different antidepressant or consider a brief period of concomitant treatment with a benzodiazepine followed by a clinical review within 2 weeks.
- St John's wort may be of benefit in mild or moderate depression, but its use should not be prescribed or advised because of uncertainty about appropriate doses, variation in the nature of preparations, and potential serious interactions with other drugs.
- Tell patients taking St John's wort about the different potencies of the preparations available and the uncertainty that arises from this, and about the interactions of St John's wort with other drugs (including oral contraceptives, anticoagulants and anticonvulsants).

Stopping or reducing antidepressants
- Inform patients about the possibility of discontinuation/withdrawal symptoms on stopping, reducing or missing doses. These symptoms are usually mild and self-limiting but can occasionally be severe, particularly if the drug is stopped abruptly.
- Advise patients to take their drugs as prescribed, particularly drugs with a shorter half-life (such as paroxetine and venlafaxine).
- Reduce doses gradually over a 4-week period; some people may require longer periods, and fluoxetine can usually be stopped over a shorter period.
- For mild discontinuation/withdrawal symptoms, reassure the patient and monitor symptoms.
- For severe symptoms, consider reintroducing the original antidepressant at the effective dose (or another antidepressant with a longer half-life from the same class) and reduce gradually while monitoring symptoms.
- Ask patients to seek advice from their medical practitioner if they experience significant discontinuation/withdrawal symptoms.

Pharmacological treatment of atypical depression
- Treat patients with features of atypical depression with an SSRI.
- If there is no response to an SSRI and there is significant functional impairment, consider referral to a mental health specialist.

Special patient characteristics

Age
- For older adults with depression, give antidepressant treatment at an age-appropriate dose for a minimum of 6 weeks before considering that it is ineffective. If there is a partial response within this period, treatment should be continued for a further 6 weeks.
- When prescribing antidepressants for older adults, consider:
  – the increased risk of drug interactions
  – careful monitoring of side effects, particularly with tricyclic antidepressants.

Patients with dementia
- Treat depression in people with dementia in the same way as depression in other older adults.

Gender
- Note that women have a poorer toleration of imipramine.

Patients with cardiovascular disease
- When initiating antidepressant treatment in patients with recent myocardial infarction or unstable angina, sertraline is the treatment of choice and has the best evidence base.
- Perform an ECG and measure blood pressure before prescribing a tricyclic antidepressant for a depressed patient at significant risk of cardiovascular disease.
- Do not prescribe venlafaxine or a tricyclic antidepressant (except lofepramine) for patients with a high risk of serious cardiac arrhythmias or recent myocardial infarction.

Limited response to initial treatment in moderate and severe depression

Pharmacological approaches
- When a patient fails to respond to the first antidepressant prescribed, check that the drug has been taken regularly and at the prescribed dose.
- If response to a standard dose of an antidepressant is inadequate, and there are no significant side effects, consider a gradual increase in dose in line with the schedule suggested by the Summary of Product Characteristics.
- Consider switching to another antidepressant if there has been no response after a month. If there has been a partial response, a decision to switch can be postponed until 6 weeks have passed.
- If an antidepressant has not been effective or is poorly tolerated and, after considering a range of other treatment options, the decision is made to offer a further course of antidepressants, then switch to another single antidepressant.
- Choices for a second antidepressant include a different SSRI or mirtazapine; alternatives include moclobemide, reboxetine and lofepramine. Consider other tricyclic antidepressants (except dosulepin) and venlafaxine, especially for more severe depression. (See notes below about switching.)
- When switching from one antidepressant to another, be aware of the need for gradual and modest incremental increases of dose, of interactions between antidepressants, and the risk of serotonin syndrome when combinations of serotonergic antidepressants are prescribed. Features include confusion, delirium, shivering, sweating, changes in blood pressure and myoclonus.

Depression 3

Limited response to initial treatment in moderate and severe depression (cont.)

Special considerations when switching to mirtazapine, moclobemide or reboxetine

- If switching to mirtazapine, be aware that it can cause sedation and weight gain.
- If switching to moclobemide, be aware of the need to wash out previously prescribed antidepressants.
- If switching to reboxetine, be aware of the relative lack of data on its side effects, and monitor carefully.

Psychological treatments

- CBT is the psychological treatment of choice. Consider interpersonal psychotherapy (IPT) if the patient expresses a preference for it or if you think the patient may benefit from it.
- CBT and IPT should be delivered by a healthcare professional competent in their use. Treatment typically consists of 16 to 20 sessions over 6 to 9 months.
- Consider CBT (or IPT) for patients with moderate or severe depression who do not take or refuse antidepressant treatment.
- For patients who have not made an adequate response to other treatments for depression (for example, antidepressants and brief psychological interventions), consider giving a course of CBT of 16 to 20 sessions over 6 to 9 months.
- Consider CBT for patients with severe depression for whom avoiding the side effects often associated with antidepressants is a clinical priority or personal preference.
- For patients with severe depression, consider providing 2 sessions of CBT per week for the first month of treatment.
- Where patients have responded to a course of individual CBT or IPT, consider offering follow-up sessions – typically 2 to 4 sessions over 12 months.

Couple-focused therapy

- Consider couple-focused therapy for people with depression who have a regular partner and who have not benefited from a brief individual intervention. An adequate course is 15 to 20 sessions over 5 to 6 months.

Special considerations when switching to a new tricyclic antidepressant

- Consider their poorer tolerability compared with other equally effective antidepressants, and the increased risk of cardiotoxicity and toxicity in overdose.
- Start on a low dose and, if there is a clear clinical response, maintain on that dose with careful monitoring.
- Gradually increase dose if there is lack of efficacy and no major side effects.
- Lofrepramine is a reasonable choice because of its relative lack of cardiotoxicity.

Special considerations when switching to venlafaxine

- Before prescribing:
  - take into account the increased likelihood of patients stopping treatment because of side effects, and its higher cost, compared with equally effective SSRIs.
  - ensure pre-existing hypertension is controlled in line with the current NICE guideline (www.nice.org.uk/CG034).
- Do not prescribe for patients with uncontrolled hypertension.
- Venlafaxine should only be prescribed at 300 mg per day or more under the supervision or advice of a specialist mental health medical practitioner.
- *Monitoring:*
  - measure blood pressure at initiation and regularly during treatment (particularly during dosage titration); reduce the dose or consider discontinuation if there is a sustained increase in blood pressure.
  - check for signs and symptoms of cardiac dysfunction, particularly in people with known cardiovascular disease, and take appropriate action as necessary.

Initial presentation of severe depression

- When patients present initially with severe depression, a combination of antidepressants and individual CBT should be considered as it is more cost-effective than either treatment on its own.

Chronic depression

- In chronic depression, offer a combination of individual CBT and antidepressant medication.
- For men with chronic depression who have not responded to an SSRI, consider a tricyclic antidepressant, as men tolerate the side effects of tricyclic antidepressants reasonably well.
- Consider offering befriending to people with chronic depression (by trained volunteers offering weekly meetings for 2 to 6 months) as an adjunct to pharmacological or psychological treatments.
- Consider a rehabilitation programme for patients who are unemployed or have been disengaged from social activities over a longer term.

Enhanced care in primary care

- For all patients, consider telephone support from the primary care team, informed by clear treatment protocols, particularly for monitoring antidepressant medication regimes.
- Primary care organisations should consider establishing multi-faceted care programmes which integrate through clearly specified protocols the delivery and monitoring of appropriate psychological and pharmacological interventions for the care of people with depression.

Depression references

These guidelines are an extract from:
National Institute for Health and Clinical Excellence. *Management of Depression in Primary and Secondary Care: NICE guideline 23*. London: NICE; 2004. Available at: www.nice.org.uk/CG23
Reproduced with permission.

Butler R, Carney S, Cipriani A, *et al*. Depressive disorders. *Clinical Evidence*. 2005; **15**: 316–68

Churchill R, Hunot V, Corney R, *et al*. A systematic review of controlled trials of the effectiveness and cost-effectiveness of brief psychological treatments for depression. *Health Technol Assess*. 2001; **5**(35): 1–173.

Department of Health. *National Service Framework for Mental Health*. London: DH; 1999. Available at: www.dh.gov.uk/en/Publicationsandstatistics/Publications/PublicationsPolicyAndGuidance/DH_4009598

Geddes JR, Carney SM, Davies C, *et al*. Relapse prevention with antidepressant drug treatment in depressive disorders: a systematic review. *Lancet*. 2003; **361**(9358): 653–61.

Gelenberg AJ, Hopkins HS. Assessing and treating depression in primary care medicine [review]. *Am J Med*. 2007; **120**(2): 105–8.

Hollon SD, DeRubeis RJ, Shelton RC, *et al*. Prevention of relapse following cognitive therapy vs medications in moderate to severe depression. *Arch Gen Psychiatry*. 2005; **62**(4): 417–22.

Lurie SJ, Gawinski B, Pierce D, *et al*. Seasonal affective disorder [review]. *Am Fam Physician*. 2006; **74**(9): 1521–4.

Scottish Intercollegiate Guidelines Network. *Postnatal Depression and Puerperal Psychosis*. Edinburgh: SIGN; 2002. Available at: www.sign.ac.uk/pdf/qrg60.pdf

Stein RE, Zitner LE, Jensen PS. Interventions for adolescent depression in primary care [review]. *Pediatrics*. 2006; **118**(2): 669–82.

8

DIABETES

WHO biochemical criteria (venous plasma) for the diagnosis of diabetes, impaired glucose tolerance and impaired fasting glycaemia or impaired fasting glucose

	Glucose concentration mmol/l (mg/dl) (venous plasma)
Diabetes mellitus	
Fasting *and/or* 2-h post-glucose load	≥7.0 (≥126) *and* ≥11.1 (≥200)
Impaired glucose tolerance (IGT)	
Fasting (if measured) *and* 2-h post-glucose load	<7.0 (<126) *and* ≥7.8 (≥140) and <11.1 (<200)
Impaired fasting glycaemia or impaired fasting glucose (IFG)	
Fasting *and (if measured)* 2-h post-glucose load	≥6.1 (≥110) and <7.0 (<126) *and (if measured)* <7.8 (<140)

From: World Health Organization. *Definition, Diagnosis and Classification of Diabetes Mellitus and its Complications.* WHO; 1999.

Blood glucose-lowering therapy

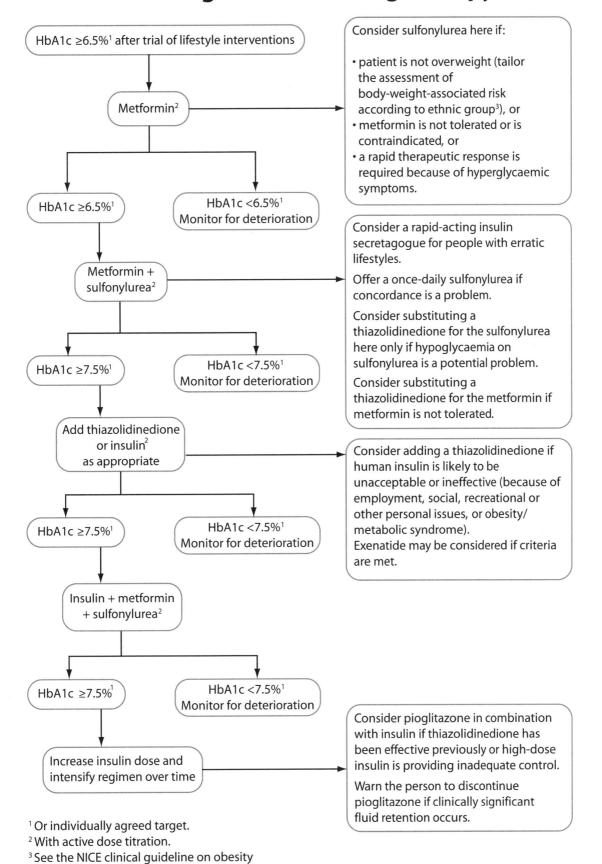

HbA1c ≥6.5%[1] after trial of lifestyle interventions

Metformin[2]

Consider sulfonylurea here if:

- patient is not overweight (tailor the assessment of body-weight-associated risk according to ethnic group[3]), or
- metformin is not tolerated or is contraindicated, or
- a rapid therapeutic response is required because of hyperglycaemic symptoms.

HbA1c ≥6.5%[1]

HbA1c <6.5%[1]
Monitor for deterioration

Metformin + sulfonylurea[2]

Consider a rapid-acting insulin secretagogue for people with erratic lifestyles.

Offer a once-daily sulfonylurea if concordance is a problem.

Consider substituting a thiazolidinedione for the sulfonylurea here only if hypoglycaemia on sulfonylurea is a potential problem.

Consider substituting a thiazolidinedione for the metformin if metformin is not tolerated.

HbA1c ≥7.5%[1]

HbA1c <7.5%[1]
Monitor for deterioration

Add thiazolidinedione or insulin[2] as appropriate

Consider adding a thiazolidinedione if human insulin is likely to be unacceptable or ineffective (because of employment, social, recreational or other personal issues, or obesity/metabolic syndrome).
Exenatide may be considered if criteria are met.

HbA1c ≥7.5%[1]

HbA1c <7.5%[1]
Monitor for deterioration

Insulin + metformin + sulfonylurea[2]

HbA1c ≥7.5%[1]

HbA1c <7.5%[1]
Monitor for deterioration

Increase insulin dose and intensify regimen over time

Consider pioglitazone in combination with insulin if thiazolidinedione has been effective previously or high-dose insulin is providing inadequate control.

Warn the person to discontinue pioglitazone if clinically significant fluid retention occurs.

[1] Or individually agreed target.
[2] With active dose titration.
[3] See the NICE clinical guideline on obesity (www.nice.org.uk/CG043).

Management of blood lipids

Review CV risk status annually:

- assess risk factors, including features of metabolic syndrome and waist circumference
- note changes in personal or family CV history
- perform full lipid profile (including HDL-C and TG) – also perform after diagnosis and repeat before starting lipid-modifying therapy.

If history of elevated serum TG, perform full fasting lipid profile (including HDL-C and TG).

Consider to be at high CV risk unless all of the following apply:

- not overweight (tailor with body-weight-associated risk assessment according to ethnic group)
- normotensive (<140/80 mmHg in absence of antihypertensive therapy)
- no microalbuminuria
- non-smoker
- no high-risk lipid profile
- no history of CV disease
- no family history of CV disease.

Estimate CV risk from UKPDS risk engine annually if assessed as not at high CV risk (see www.dtu.ox.ac.uk/index.php?maindoc=/riskengine/).

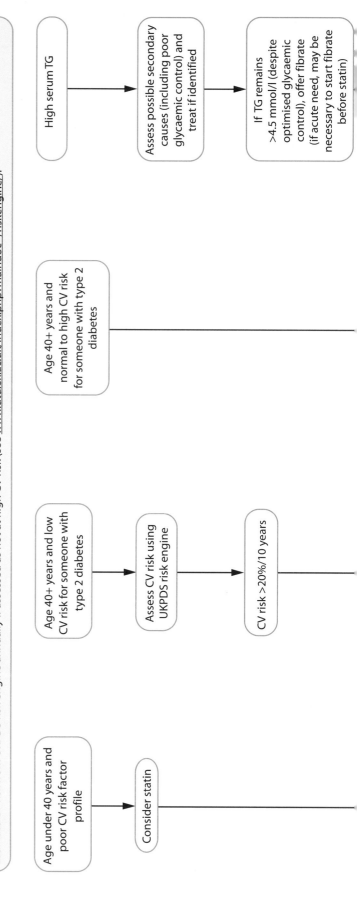

High serum TG

↓

Assess possible secondary causes (including poor glycaemic control) and treat if identified

↓

If TG remains >4.5 mmol/l (despite optimised glycaemic control), offer fibrate (if acute need, may be necessary to start fibrate before statin)

Age 40+ years and normal to high CV risk for someone with type 2 diabetes

Age 40+ years and low CV risk for someone with type 2 diabetes

↓

Assess CV risk using UKPDS risk engine

↓

CV risk >20%/10 years

Age under 40 years and poor CV risk factor profile

↓

Consider statin

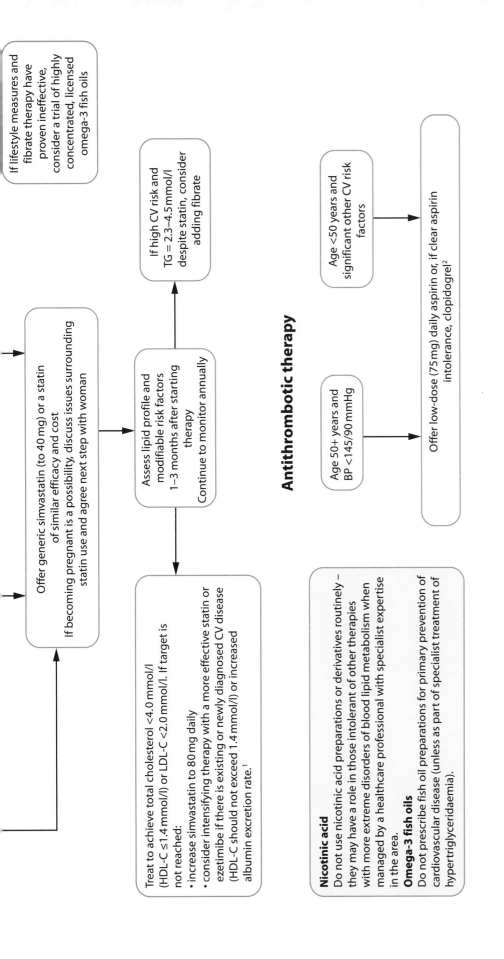

If lifestyle measures and fibrate therapy have proven ineffective, consider a trial of highly concentrated, licensed omega-3 fish oils

Offer generic simvastatin (to 40 mg) or a statin of similar efficacy and cost

If becoming pregnant is a possibility, discuss issues surrounding statin use and agree next step with woman

Assess lipid profile and modifiable risk factors
1–3 months after starting therapy
Continue to monitor annually

If high CV risk and TG = 2.3–4.5 mmol/l despite statin, consider adding fibrate

Treat to achieve total cholesterol <4.0 mmol/l (HDL-C ≤1.4 mmol/l) or LDL-C <2.0 mmol/l. If target is not reached:
• increase simvastatin to 80 mg daily
• consider intensifying therapy with a more effective statin or ezetimibe if there is existing or newly diagnosed CV disease (HDL-C should not exceed 1.4 mmol/l) or increased albumin excretion rate.[1]

Nicotinic acid
Do not use nicotinic acid preparations or derivatives routinely – they may have a role in those intolerant of other therapies with more extreme disorders of blood lipid metabolism when managed by a healthcare professional with specialist expertise in the area.

Omega-3 fish oils
Do not prescribe fish oil preparations for primary prevention of cardiovascular disease (unless as part of specialist treatment of hypertriglyceridaemia).

Antithrombotic therapy

Age 50+ years and BP <145/90 mmHg

Age <50 years and significant other CV risk factors

Offer low-dose (75 mg) daily aspirin or, if clear aspirin intolerance, clopidogrel[2]

CV = cardiovascular; HDL–C = high-density lipoprotein–cholesterol; LDL–C = low-density lipoprotein–cholesterol; TG = triglyceride; BP = blood pressure.

[1] National Institute for Health and Clinical Excellence (NICE). *Statins for the Prevention of Cardiovascular Events in Patients at Increased Risk of Developing Cardiovascular Disease or Those with Established Cardiovascular Disease: NICE technology appraisal 94.* London: NICE; 2006. NICE. *Ezetimibe for the Treatment of Primary (heterozygous-familial and non-familial) Hypercholesterolaemia: NICE technology appraisal 132.* London: NICE; 2005.

[2] NICE. *Clopidogrel and Modified-Release Dipyridamole in the Prevention of Occlusive Vascular Events: NICE technology appraisal 90.* London: NICE; 2005.

Blood pressure management

Targets
- If kidney, eye or cerebrovascular damage, set a target <130/80 mmHg.
- Others, set a target <140/80 mmHg.

If on antihypertensive therapy at diagnosis of diabetes:
- review BP control and medication use
- make changes only if BP is poorly controlled or current medications are inappropriate because of microvascular complications or metabolic problems.

If the person's BP reaches and consistently remains at the target:
- monitor every 4–6 months and check for possible adverse effects of antihypertensive therapy (including those from unnecessarily low blood pressure).

Measure BP annually if not hypertensive or with renal disease.
If BP > target, repeat measurement within:
- 1 month if >150/90 mmHg
- 2 months if >140/80 mmHg
- 2 months if >130/80 mmHg and kidney, eye or cerebrovascular damage

BP above target

Advise on lifestyle measures
Dietary advice and see NICE clinical guideline on hypertension (www.nice.org.uk/CG034)

BP above target

Offer ACE inhibitor (titrate dose)
For people of African-Caribbean descent, offer ACE inhibitor plus diuretic or CCB

> If there is a possibility of the person becoming pregnant, start with a CCB.
> If continuing intolerance to ACE inhibitor (other than renal deterioration or hyperkalaemia), change to an A2RB.

BP above target

Add CCB or diuretic
(usually bendroflumethiazide, 2.5 mg daily)

BP above target

Add other drug (diuretic or CCB – see above)

BP above target

Add alpha blocker, beta blocker or potassium-sparing diuretic

> Use a potassium-sparing diuretic with caution if already taking ACE inhibitor or A2RB.

Maintain lifestyle measures

Monitor BP 1–2 monthly until consistently below target

Antihypertensive medications can increase the likelihood of side effects such as orthostatic hypotension in a person with autonomic neuropathy.

A2RB = angiotensin II receptor blocker; AER = albumin excretion rate; BP = blood pressure; CCB = calcium-channel blocker.

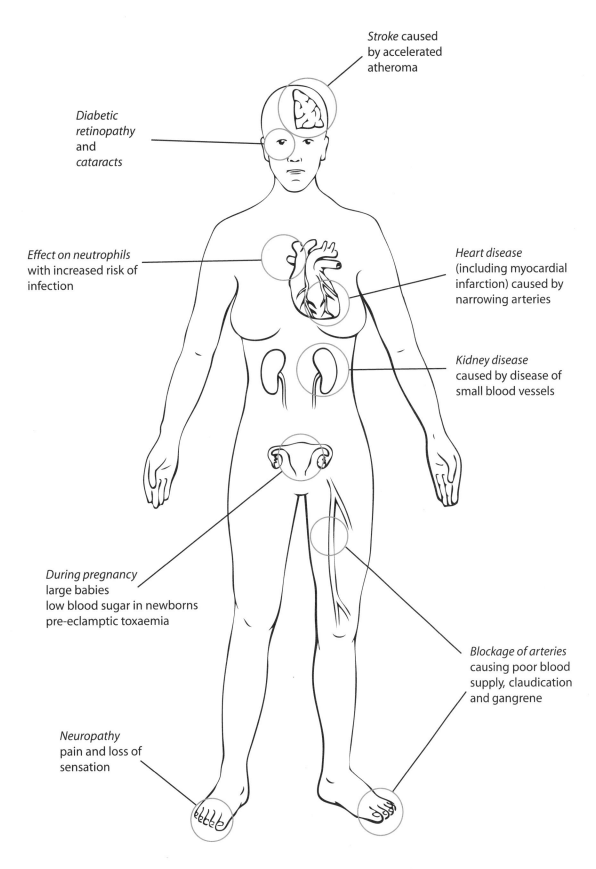

Stroke caused by accelerated atheroma

Diabetic retinopathy and cataracts

Effect on neutrophils with increased risk of infection

Heart disease (including myocardial infarction) caused by narrowing arteries

Kidney disease caused by disease of small blood vessels

During pregnancy large babies low blood sugar in newborns pre-eclamptic toxaemia

Blockage of arteries causing poor blood supply, claudication and gangrene

Neuropathy pain and loss of sensation

Figure 8.1 The major complications of diabetes

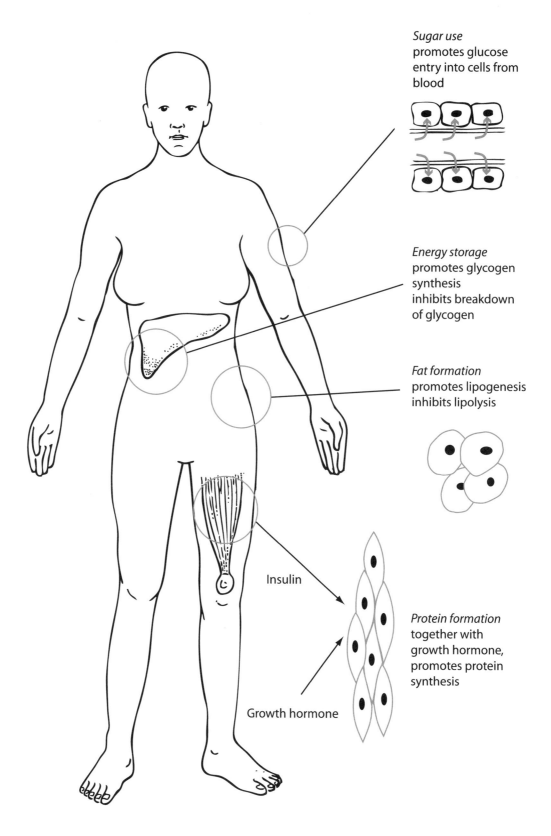

Sugar use
promotes glucose
entry into cells from
blood

Energy storage
promotes glycogen
synthesis
inhibits breakdown
of glycogen

Fat formation
promotes lipogenesis
inhibits lipolysis

Insulin

Growth hormone

Protein formation
together with
growth hormone,
promotes protein
synthesis

Figure 8.2 Important actions of insulin

Diabetes references

The blood glucose control, lipid control and blood pressure control in diabetes are extracts from the following guideline:

National Institute for Health and Clinical Excellence. *The Management of Type 2 Diabetes: NICE guideline 66*. London: NICE; 2008. Available at: www.nice.org. uk/CG66

Reproduced with permission.

Action to Control Cardiovascular Risk in Diabetes (ACCORD) Study Group. Effects of intensive glucose lowering in type 2 diabetes. *N Engl J Med*. 2008; **358**(24): 2545–59.

ADVANCE Collaborative Group. Intensive blood glucose control and vascular outcomes in patients with type 2 diabetes. *N Engl J Med*. 2008; **358**(24): 2560–72.

Campbell A. Glycaemic control in type 2 diabetes. *BMJ Clinical Evidence*. 2005; **4** (14); 474–90

Department of Health. *National Service Framework for Diabetes*. London: DH; 2003. Available at: www.dh.gov.uk/en/Publicationsandstatistics/Pressreleases/ DH_4079940

Garber AJ. Benefits of combination therapy of insulin and oral hypoglycemic agents. *Arch Intern Med*. 2003; **163**(15): 1781–2.

Owens D, Barnett AH, Pickup J, *et al*. Blood glucose self-monitoring in type 1 and type 2 diabetes: reaching a multidisciplinary consensus. *Diabetes and Primary Care*. 2004; **6**(1): 8–19.

Raleigh VS. Diabetes and hypertension in Britain's ethnic minorities: implications for the future of renal services [review]. *BMJ*. 1997; **314**(7075): 209–13.

Rendell M. The role of sulphonylureas in the management of type 2 diabetes mellitus. *Drugs*. 2004; **64**(12): 1339–58.

Reynolds TM, Smellie WS, Twomey PJ. Glycated haemoglobin (HbA1c) monitoring. *BMJ*. 2006; **333**(7568): 586–8.

World Health Organization. *Definition, Diagnosis and Classification of Diabetes Mellitus and its Complications: Part 1: diagnosis and classification of diabetes mellitus provisional report of a WHO consultation*. Geneva: WHO; 1999. Available at: www.diabetes.com.au/pdf/who_report.pdf

9

DYSPEPSIA

Presentation at GP and endoscopy
Flowchart of referral criteria and subsequent management

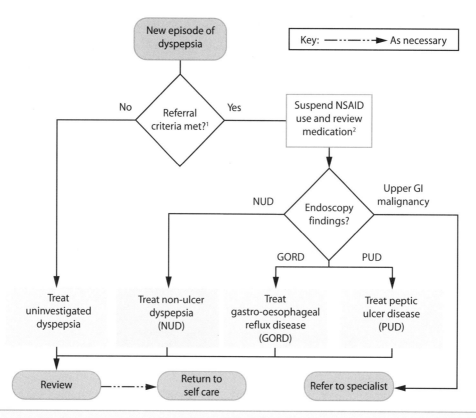

1 Immediate referral is indicated for significant acute gastrointestinal bleeding.
Consider the possibility of cardiac or biliary disease as part of the differential diagnosis.
Urgent* specialist referral for endoscopic investigation is indicated for patients of any age with dyspepsia when presenting with any of the following: chronic gastrointestinal bleeding, progressive unintentional weight loss, progressive difficulty swallowing, persistent vomiting, iron deficiency anaemia, epigastric mass or suspicious barium meal.

Routine endoscopic investigation of patients of any age presenting with dyspepsia and without alarm signs is not necessary. However, in patients aged 55 years and older with unexplained** and persistent** recent-onset dyspepsia alone, an urgent referral for endoscopy should be made.

Consider managing previously investigated patients without new alarm signs according to previous endoscopic findings.

2 Review medications for possible causes of dyspepsia, for example, calcium antagonists, nitrates, theophyllines, bisphosphonates, steroids and NSAIDs. Patients undergoing endoscopy should be free from medication with either a proton pump inhibitor (PPI) or an H2 receptor (H2RA) for a minimum of 2 weeks.

* The Guideline Development Group considered that 'urgent' meant being seen within 2 weeks.
** In the referral guidelines for suspected cancer (*NICE guideline 27*), 'unexplained' is defined as 'a symptom(s) and/or sign(s) that has not led to a diagnosis being made by the primary care professional after initial assessment of the history, examination and primary care investigations (if any)'. In the context of this recommendation, the primary care professional should confirm that the dyspepsia is new rather than a recurrent episode and exclude common precipitants of dyspepsia such as ingestion of NSAIDs. 'Persistent' as used in the recommendations in the referral guidelines refers to the continuation of specified symptoms and/or signs beyond a period that would normally be associated with self-limiting problems.

The precise period will vary depending on the severity of symptoms and associated features, as assessed by the health-care professional. In many cases, the upper limit the professional will permit symptoms and/or signs to persist before initiating referral will be 4–6 weeks.

Management flowchart for patients with uninvestigated dyspepsia

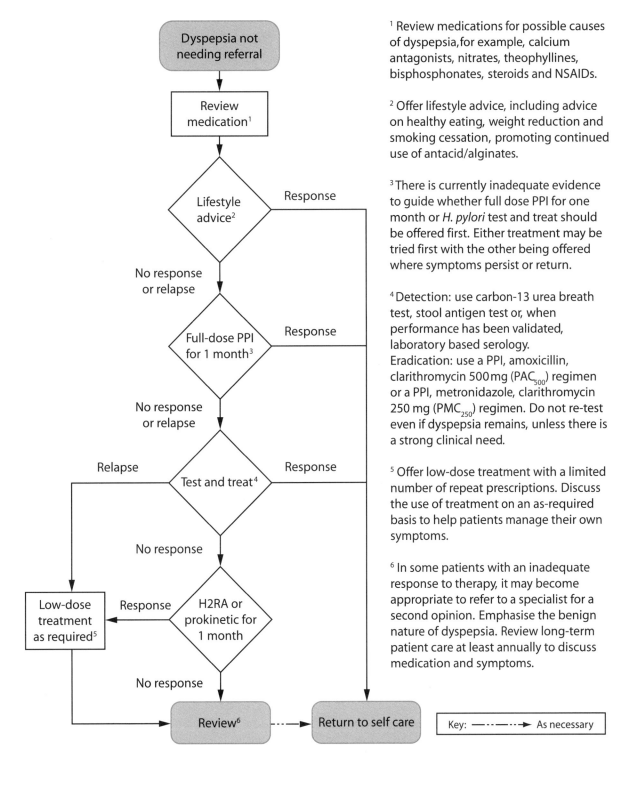

¹ Review medications for possible causes of dyspepsia, for example, calcium antagonists, nitrates, theophyllines, bisphosphonates, steroids and NSAIDs.

² Offer lifestyle advice, including advice on healthy eating, weight reduction and smoking cessation, promoting continued use of antacid/alginates.

³ There is currently inadequate evidence to guide whether full dose PPI for one month or *H. pylori* test and treat should be offered first. Either treatment may be tried first with the other being offered where symptoms persist or return.

⁴ Detection: use carbon-13 urea breath test, stool antigen test or, when performance has been validated, laboratory based serology.
Eradication: use a PPI, amoxicillin, clarithromycin 500 mg (PAC$_{500}$) regimen or a PPI, metronidazole, clarithromycin 250 mg (PMC$_{250}$) regimen. Do not re-test even if dyspepsia remains, unless there is a strong clinical need.

⁵ Offer low-dose treatment with a limited number of repeat prescriptions. Discuss the use of treatment on an as-required basis to help patients manage their own symptoms.

⁶ In some patients with an inadequate response to therapy, it may become appropriate to refer to a specialist for a second opinion. Emphasise the benign nature of dyspepsia. Review long-term patient care at least annually to discuss medication and symptoms.

Reviewing patient care

Recommendations

- Offer patients requiring long-term management of dyspepsia symptoms an annual review of their condition, encouraging them to try stepping down or stopping treatment.*

- A return to self-treatment with antacid and/or alginate therapy (either prescribed or purchased over the counter and taken as required) may be appropriate.

- Offer simple lifestyle advice, including healthy eating, weight reduction and smoking cessation.

- Advise patients to avoid known precipitants they associate with their dyspepsia where possible. These include smoking, alcohol, coffee, chocolate, fatty foods and being overweight. Raising the head of the bed and having a main meal well before going to bed may help some people.

- Routine endoscopic investigation of patients of any age, presenting with dyspepsia and without alarm signs, is not necessary. However, in patients aged 55 years and older with unexplained** and persistent** recent-onset dyspepsia alone, an urgent referral for endoscopy should be made.

* Unless there is an underlying condition or co-medication requiring continuing treatment.
** In the referral guidelines for suspected cancer (*NICE guideline 27*), 'unexplained' is defined as 'a symptom(s) and/or sign(s) that has not led to a diagnosis being made by the primary care professional after initial assessment of the history, examination and primary care investigations (if any)'. In the context of this recommendation, the primary care professional should confirm that the dyspepsia is new rather than a recurrent episode and exclude common precipitants of dyspepsia such as ingestion of NSAIDs. 'Persistent' as used in the recommendations in the referral guidelines refers to the continuation of specified symptoms and/or signs beyond a period that would normally be associated with self-limiting problems. The precise period will vary depending on the severity of symptoms and associated features, as assessed by the healthcare professional. In many cases, the upper limit the professional will permit symptoms and/or signs to persist before initiating referral will be 4–6 weeks.

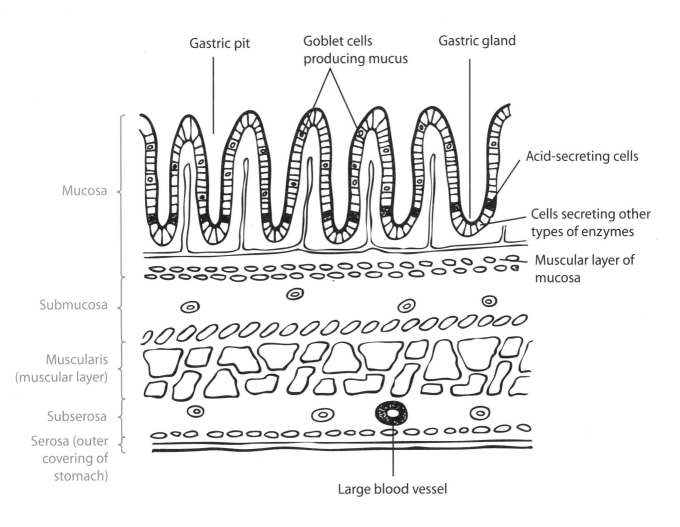

Figure 9.1 Structure of stomach wall

Dyspepsia references

These guidelines are an extract from:
National Institute for Health and Clinical Excellence. *Management of Dyspepsia in Adults in Primary Care: NICE guideline 17*. London: NICE; 2005. Available at: www.nice.org.uk/CG17
Reproduced with permission.

Bardhan KD. Intermittent and on-demand use of proton pump inhibitors in the management of symptomatic gastroesophageal reflux disease. *Am J Gastroenterol*. 2003; **98**(Suppl. 3): S40–8.

British Society of Gastroenterology. *Dyspepsia Management Guidelines*. London: BSG; 2002. Available at: www.bsg.org.uk/pdf_word_docs/dyspepsia.doc

Chiba N, Thompson ABR, Barkun AN. The Rome II definition of dyspepsia does not exclude patients with GERD in primary care. *Gastroenterology*. 2003; **124**(4, Suppl. 1): S223–4.

Delaney B, Ford A, Forman D, *et al*. Eradication therapy for peptic ulcer disease in *Helicobacter pylori* positive patients. *Cochrane Database Syst Rev*. 2006; **1**: CD003840.

Drug and Therapeutics Bulletin. The medical management of gastro-oesophageal reflux. *Drug Ther Bull*. 1996; **34**(1): 1–4.

Malfertheiner P, Megraud F, O'Morain C, *et al*. Current concepts in the management of *Helicobacter pylori* infection – the Maastricht 2-2000 consensus report. *Aliment Pharmacol Ther*. 2002; **16**(2): 167–80.

Meurer LN, Bower DJ. Management of *Helicobacter pylori* infection. *Am Fam Physician*. 2002; **65**(7): 1327–36.

National Institute for Health and Clinical Excellence. *Referral Guidelines for Suspected Cancer: quick reference guide: NICE guideline 27*. London: NICE; 2005. Available at: www.nice.org.uk/Guidance/CG27 (summarised in this book).

Scottish Intercollegiate Guideline Network. *Dyspepsia: SIGN guideline 68*. Edinburgh: SIGN; 2003. Available at: www.sign.ac.uk/pdf/sign68.pdf

Uemura N, Okamoto S, Yamamoto S, *et al*. *Helicobacter pylori* infection and the development of gastric cancer. *New Engl J Med*. 2001; **345**(11): 784–9.

Management flowchart for patients with non-ulcer dyspepsia

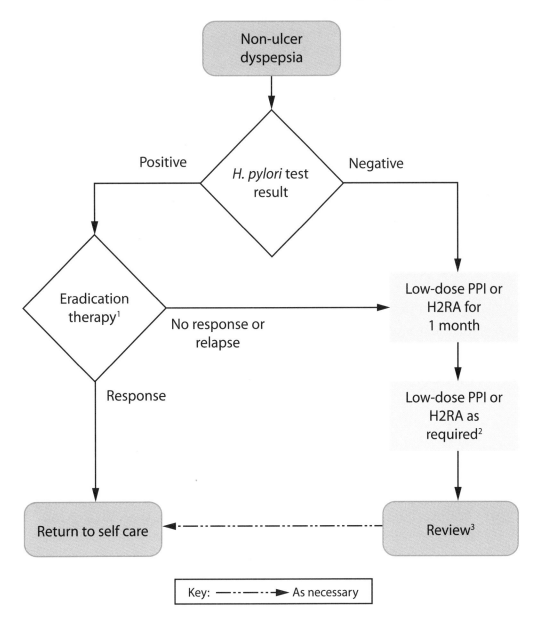

Non-ulcer dyspepsia

H. pylori test result

Positive

Negative

Eradication therapy[1]

Low-dose PPI or H2RA for 1 month

No response or relapse

Response

Low-dose PPI or H2RA as required[2]

Return to self care

Review[3]

Key: ———·—·—·—► As necessary

1 Use a PPI, amoxicillin, clarithromycin 500mg (PAC$_{500}$) regimen or a PPI, metronidazole, clarithromycin 250mg (PMC$_{250}$) regimen. Do not re-test unless there is a strong clinical need.

2 Offer low-dose treatment, possibly on an as-required basis, with a limited number of repeat prescriptions.

3 In some patients with an inadequate response to therapy or new emergent symptoms, it may become appropriate to refer to a specialist for a second opinion. Emphasise the benign nature of dyspepsia. Review long-term patient care at least annually through discussion of medication and symptoms with patient.

Non-ulcer dyspepsia references

This guideline is an extract from:

National Institute for Health and Clinical Excellence. *Management of Dyspepsia in Adults in Primary Care: NICE guideline 17*. London: NICE; 2005. Available at: www.nice.org.uk/CG17

Reproduced with permission.

Delaney BC, Moayyedi P, Forman D. Initial management strategies for dyspepsia. *Cochrane Database Syst Rev*. 2003; **2**: CD001961.

Drug and Therapeutics Bulletin. Which test for *Helicobacter pylori* in primary care? *Drug Ther Bull*. 2004; **42**(9): 71–2.

Ford AC, Qume M, Moayyedi P, *et al*. Helicobacter pylori 'test and treat' or endoscopy for managing dyspepsia: an individual patient data meta-analysis. *Gastroenterology*. 2005; **128**(7): 1838–44.

Kligler B, Chaudhary S. Peppermint oil [review]. *Am Fam Physician*. 2007; **75**(7): 1027–30.

Malfertheiner P, Megraud F, O'Morain C, *et al*. Current concepts in the management of *Helicobacter pylori* infection: the Maastricht III Consensus Report. *Gut*. 2007; **56**(6): 772–81.

Mazzoleni LE, Sander GB, Ott EA, *et al*. Clinical outcomes of eradication of *Helicobacter pylori* in non-ulcer dyspepsia in a population with a high prevalence of infection: results of a 12-month randomized, double blind, placebo-controlled study. *Dig Dis Sci*. 2006; **51**(1): 89–98.

National Institute for Health and Clinical Excellence. *Referral for Suspected Cancer: quick reference guide: NICE guideline 27*. London: NICE; 2005. Available at: www.nice.org.uk/CG27

Peura DA, Gudmundson J, Siepman N, *et al*. Proton pump inhibitors: effective first-line treatment for management of dyspepsia. *Dig Dis Sci*. 2007; **52**(4): 983–7.

Scottish Intercollegiate Guideline Network. *Dyspepsia: SIGN guideline 68*. Edinburgh: SIGN; 2003. Available at: www.sign.ac.uk/pdf/qrg68.pdf

Shah R. Dyspepsia and *Helicobacter pylori* [review]. *BMJ*. 2007; **334**(7583): 41–3.

Management flowchart for patients with GORD

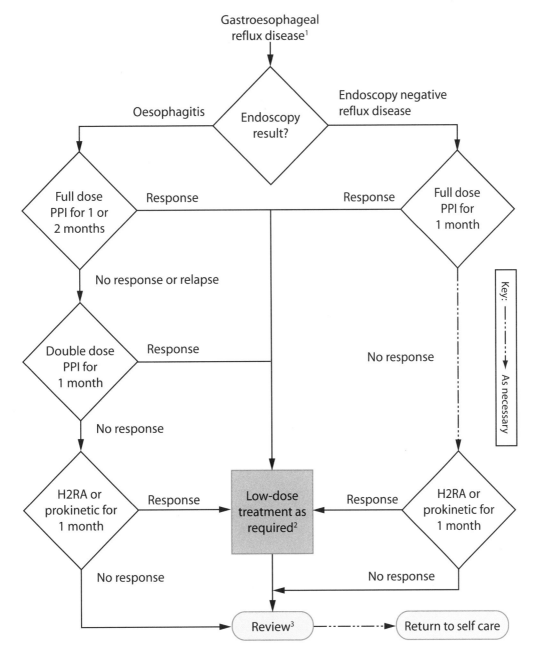

Gastroesophageal reflux disease[1]

Endoscopy result?

Oesophagitis

Endoscopy negative reflux disease

Full dose PPI for 1 or 2 months

Response

Full dose PPI for 1 month

Response

No response or relapse

Double dose PPI for 1 month

Response

No response

No response

H2RA or prokinetic for 1 month

Response

Low-dose treatment as required[2]

Response

H2RA or prokinetic for 1 month

No response

No response

Key: ⎯⎯⎯ → As necessary

Review[3] ⟶ Return to self care

1 GORD refers to endoscopically determined oesophagitis or endoscopy-negative reflux disease. Patients with uninvestigated 'reflux-like' symptoms should be managed as patients with uninvestigated dyspepsia. There is currently no evidence that *H. pylori* should be investigated in patients with GORD.

2 Offer low-dose treatment, possibly on an as-required basis, with a limited number of repeat prescriptions.

3 Review long-term patient care at least annually through discussion of medication and symptoms with patient. In some patients with an inadequate response to therapy or new emergent symptoms it may become appropriate to refer to a specialist for a second opinion.
A minority of patients have persistent symptoms despite PPI therapy, and this group remain a challenge to treat. Therapeutic options include doubling the dose of PPI therapy, adding an H2RA at bedtime and extending the length of treatment.

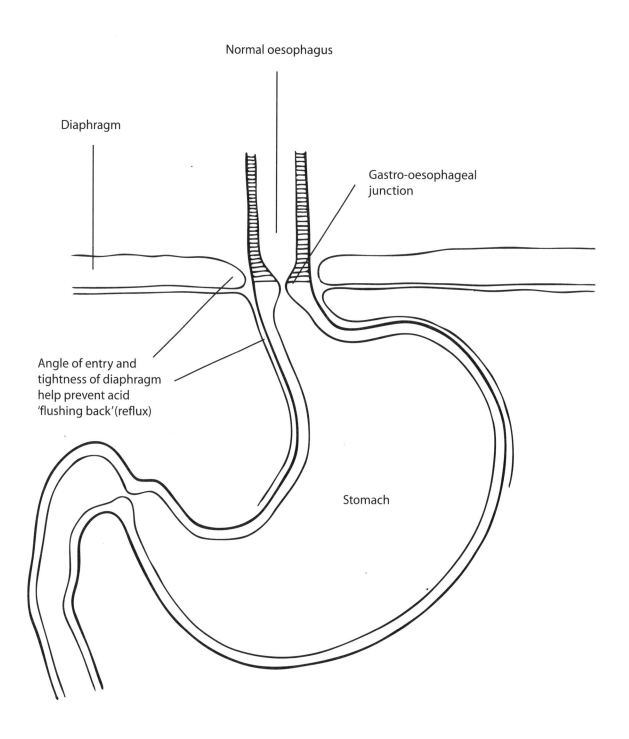

Figure 9.2 Normal stomach and oesophagus

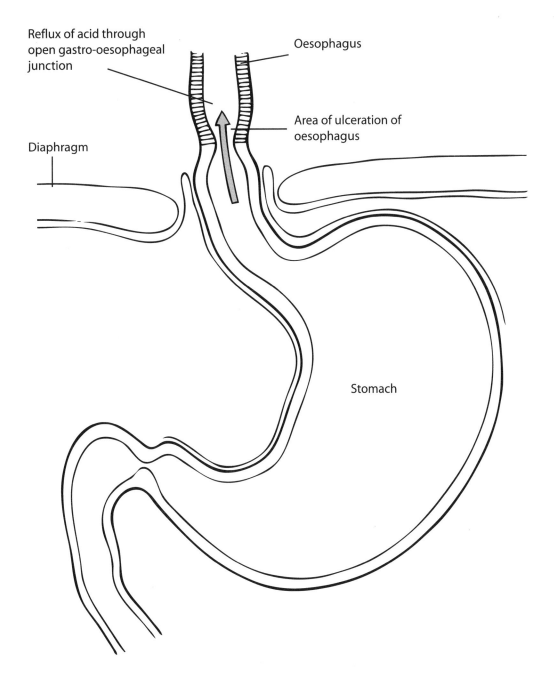

Reflux of acid through
open gastro-oesophageal
junction

Oesophagus

Area of ulceration of
oesophagus

Diaphragm

Stomach

Figure 9.3 Sliding hiatus hernia showing reflux

GORD references

These guidelines are an extract from:

National Institute for Health and Clinical Excellence. *Management of Dyspepsia in Adults in Primary Care: NICE guideline 17*. London: NICE; 2005. Available at: www.nice.org.uk/CG17

Reproduced with permission.

Bardhan KD. Intermittent and on-demand use of proton pump inhibitors in the management of symptomatic gastroesophageal reflux disease. *Am J Gastroenterol.* 2003; **98**(Suppl. 3): S40–8.

Chang JT, Katzka DA. Gastroesophageal reflux disease, Barrett esophagus, and esophageal adenocarcinoma. *Arch Intern Med.* 2004; **164**(14): 1482–8.

Delaney B, Moayyedi P. Eradicating *H. Pylori. BMJ.* 2004; **328**(7453): 1388–9

Drug & Therapeutics Bulletin. Should *H. Pylori* be eradicated in non-ulcer dyspepsia? *Drug Ther Bull.* 2002; **40**(3): 23–4.

Edwards SJ, Lind T, Lundell L. Systematic review of proton pump inhibitors for the acute treatment of reflux oesophagitis. *Aliment Pharmacol Ther.* 2001; **15**(11): 1729–36.

Galmiche JP, Letessier E, Scarpignato C. Treatment of gastro-oesophageal reflux disease in adults. *BMJ.* 1998; **316**(7146): 1720–3.

Moayyedi P, Delaney B, Forman D. Gastro-oesophageal reflux disease. *BMJ Clinical Evidence.* 2006; **08**: 403.

National Institute for Health and Clinical Excellence. *Guidance on the Use of Proton Pump Inhibitors in the Treatment of Dyspepsia: NICE technology appraisal guidance 7*. London: NICE; 2000. Available at: www.nice.org.uk/guidance/index. jsp?action=article&o=32052

National Institute for Health and Clinical Excellence. *Referral Guidelines for Suspected Cancer: quick reference guide: NICE guideline 27*. London: NICE; 2005. Available at: www.nice.org.uk/nicemedia/pdf/CG027quickrefguide.pdf

Spechler SJ. Managing Barrett's oesophagus. *BMJ.* 2003; **326**(7395): 892–4.

10

ECZEMA

Eczema: widespread and localised flare-ups 1

Which therapy?

Settle inflammation with topical corticosteroids for all patients.

In adults	In children and infants

Face, genitals and flexures
• Mildly potent corticosteroid.
Eyelids
• Mildly potent corticosteroid for 14 days at most. Monitor intra-ocular pressure in people over the age of 35 years if the treatment is used frequently.
Palms, soles of the feet and scalp
• Potent corticosteroid.
Trunk and limbs
• Lowest potency of corticosteroid likely to work within 7–14 days of treatment, based upon the severity of inflammation and response to previous treatment.
• Review if there are no significant signs of improvement within 7 days, and step up to a more potent steroid.
• Alternatively, for mild to moderate eczema treat with a potent corticosteroid for 3 days (short-burst treatment).
	• Treat all skin areas with a mildly potent corticosteroid as a first choice.
	• Occasional use of moderately potent preparations on areas other than the face, genitals or flexures may be used as an alternative treatment.
	Treat visibly infected eczema with oral antibiotics
	• Flucloxacillin or erythromycin (if the person is allergic to penicillin) are first-line treatments.
	Manage frequent flare-ups
	Review and emphasise the use of emollients
	• Increase the intensity of emollient treatment, if acceptable to the person, by all or any of the following:
	  – changing the emollient to one with a higher lipid content (lotion to a cream, or a cream to an ointment)
	  – increasing the frequency of application of the emollient
	  – increasing the quantity of emollient applied.
	Review factors that might be provoking flare-ups:
	• Avoid environmental irritants or stresses.
	• Consider antigen avoidance measures if other measures fail.

Practical prescribing points

For further information please see the Medicines Compendium (www.medicines.org.uk) or the British National Formulary (www.bnf.org).

Frequency of application
• The evidence suggests that once-daily application of topical corticosteroids is as effective as more frequent application. Note that most manufacturers recommend two or three applications per day.

Give specific advice regarding the quantity of steroid to apply
• Where larger areas require treatment, explain and demonstrate the use of the fingertip unit (FTU). One FTU weighs about 500 mg. It is roughly equivalent to the amount of cream or ointment that can be squeezed from a tube with a standard nozzle onto an adult index finger from the tip of the finger to the first crease.

  – For an adult, one FTU of topical corticosteroid is sufficient to treat a skin area about twice that of the flat of the hand with the fingers.
  – For a child aged 6 months to 1 year, use a quarter of the adult amount.
  – For a child aged 1 year to 4 years, use a third of the adult amount.
• Prescribe sufficient topical corticosteroid to treat the flare-up until it is completely resolved.

Table 1 Suitable quantities of corticosteroid to prescribe for a flare-up in an adult

Body area	Amount of corticosteroid to prescribe
Face and neck	30g
Both hands	30g
Scalp	30g
Both arms	30 to 60g
Both legs	100g
Trunk	100g
Groins and genitalia	30g

Occlusion increases both the absorption and effect of topical corticosteroids. If the area affected is occluded (e.g. the nappy area), use a weaker corticosteroid.

Eczema: widespread and localised flare-ups 2

Should I refer or investigate?

Refer?

- **Disseminated herpes simplex virus infection** – arrange emergency admission for confirmation of the diagnosis and antiviral treatment.
- **Unresponsive severe disease,** including bacterially infected eczema unresponsive to treatment with oral antibiotics and topical corticosteroids – arrange emergency admission or urgent referral depending on severity.
- **Eczema requiring a duration and potency of treatment with topical corticosteroids that risks skin thinning** (i.e. if a potent corticosteroid is required on the same area of skin of the trunk or limbs on average more frequently than 7 days within a 5-week period) – the risk is increased:
    - in thin skin and flexural areas
    - with increasing duration of use
    - when corticosteroids are used with occlusion.
- **Uncontrolled eczema where dietary factors are suspected**, arrange consultation with a dietitian.
- **Where there is diagnostic uncertainty.**

In a widespread flare-up
- **Eczema requiring a duration and/or potency of treatment with topical corticosteroids that risks systemic adverse effects.**

Table 2 Weekly dose of corticosteroids unlikely to cause systemic adverse effects in adults

Treatment period (months)	Mild and moderately potent	Potent	Very potent
< 2 months	100g	50g	30g
2–6 months	50g	30g	15g
6–12 months	25g	15g	7.5g

Investigate? (localised and widespread)

Microbiological investigation is indicated to ascertain sensitivities when infected eczema does not respond to first-line antibiotics.

Follow-up advice for localised flare-ups

- Review after 7 days if the condition is not responding well to treatment.
- Review at any stage if the condition deteriorates despite treatment.

Ezcema: widespread flare-up – severe

Which therapy?

- **Exclude eczema herpeticum** – if suspected, arrange emergency admission.
- **Arrange urgent referral or emergency admission**, depending on clinical judgement, if a widespread flare-up is:
    - severe
    - not responding well to topical corticosteroids of appropriate potency
    - distressing to the person.
- **Prescribe an antibiotic** if the person is awaiting urgent referral and there are any features of infection.
- **Consider prescribing oral prednisolone** if the person is awaiting urgent referral.
- **Oral corticosteroids should be continued until the individual is seen by a specialist**, as there is a risk of rebound flare-up when stopped. It is therefore important that the person is seen within 7 days, to avoid prolonged oral steroid use.
- **Flucloxacillin or erythromycin** are first-line antibiotics.

Practical prescribing points

For further information please see the Medicines Compendium (www.medicines.org.uk) or the British National Formulary (www.bnf.org).

- Start with 30mg prednisolone once daily and reduce the dose by 5mg a day as soon as inflammation settles. Continue on the lowest dose of oral corticosteroid that manages the inflammation adequately until the specialist sees the patient.

Should I refer or investigate?

- **Seek specialist help if a widespread flare-up is**:
    - severe
    - not responding well to topical corticosteroids of appropriate potency
    - distressing to the person.
- The decision to arrange emergency admission or urgent outpatient review for someone with unresponsive severe disease will depend on clinical judgement.
- **Disseminated herpes simplex virus infection (eczema herpeticum)** is potentially life-threatening, and if suspected should prompt emergency admission for confirmation of the diagnosis and anti-viral treatment.

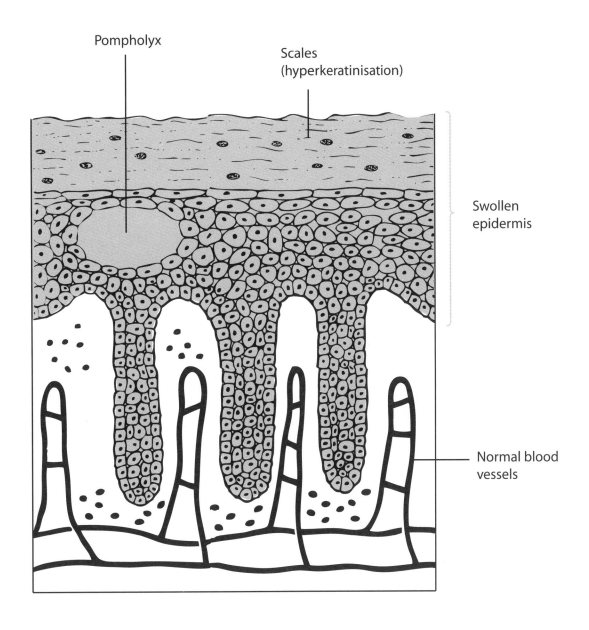

Pompholyx

Scales
(hyperkeratinisation)

Swollen
epidermis

Normal blood
vessels

Figure 10.1 Eczematous skin

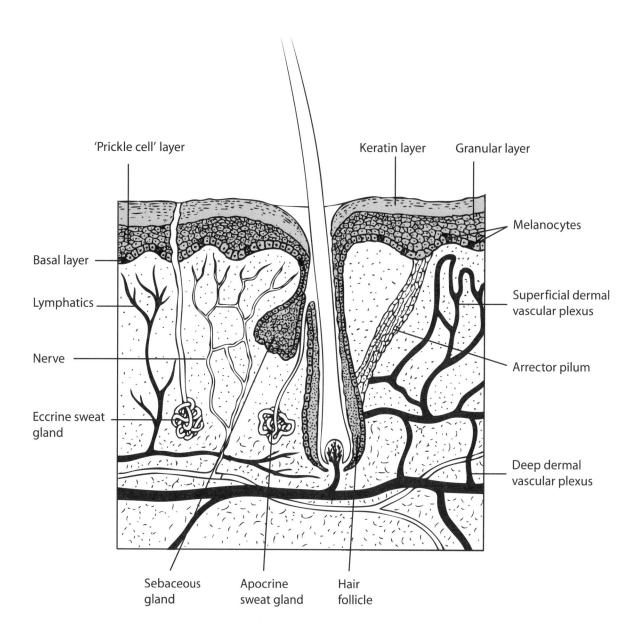

Figure 10.2 Normal epidermis

Eczema references

These guidelines are an extract from the excellent online primary care resource Clinical Knowledge Summaries, the successor to PRODIGY. Reproduced with permission. These pages are extracts from the eczema scenarios section, which is due to be revised. Please check online if in any doubt. Available at: www.cks.library.nhs.uk/eczema_atopic

Barnetson RS, Rogers M. Childhood atopic eczema. *BMJ*. 2002; **324**(7350): 1376–9.

Gdalevich M, Minouni D, David M, *et al*. Breast-feeding and the onset of atopic dermatitis in childhood: a systematic review and meta-analysis of prospective studies. *J Am Acad Dermatol*. 2001; **45**: 520–7.

Green C, Colquitt JL, Kirby J, *et al*. Clinical and cost-effectiveness of once daily versus more frequent use of same potency topical corticosteroids for atopic eczema: a systematic review and economic evaluation. *Health Technol Assess*. 2004; **8**: 1–120.

Hoare C, Li Wan Po A, Williams H. Systematic review of treatments for atopic eczema. *Health Technol Assess*. 2000; **4**:1–191.

Kay J, Gawkrodger DJ, Mortimer MJ, *et al*. The prevalence of childhood atopic eczema in a general population. *J Am Acad Dermatol*. 1994; **30**: 35–9.

Langan SM, Flohr C, Williams HC. The role of furry pets in eczema: a systematic review. *Arch Dermatol*. 2007; **143**(12): 1570–7.

Long CC, Mills CM, Finlay AY. A practical guide to topical therapy in children. *Br J Dermatol*. 1998; **138**(2): 293–6.

Tarini BA, Carroll AE, Sox CM, *et al*. Systematic review of the relationship between early introduction of solid foods to infants and the development of allergic disease. *Arch Pediatr Adolesc Med*. 2006; **160**(5): 502–7.

Weatherhead S, Robson SC, Reynolds NJ. Eczema in pregnancy [review]. *BMJ*. 2007; **335**(7611): 152–4.

Williams HC. Established corticosteroid creams should be applied only once daily in patients with atopic eczema [review]. *BMJ*. 2007; **334**(7606): 1272.

11

EPILEPSY

Epilepsy: outline care algorithm – adults

This NICE guideline is very comprehensive – the appropriate NICE quick reference guide (QRG) should be referred to for further information at each point marked with an asterisk.

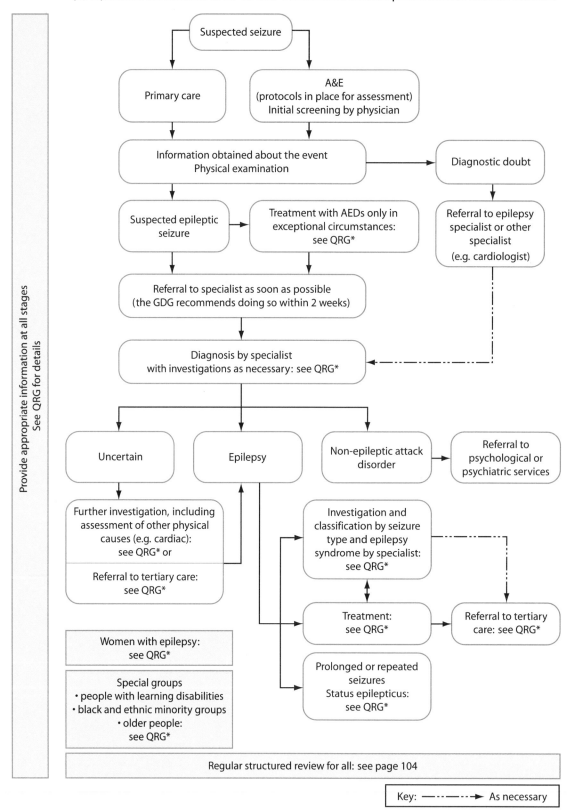

Epilepsy: outline care algorithm – children

This NICE guideline is very comprehensive – the appropriate NICE quick reference guide (QRG) should be referred to for further information at each point marked with an asterisk.

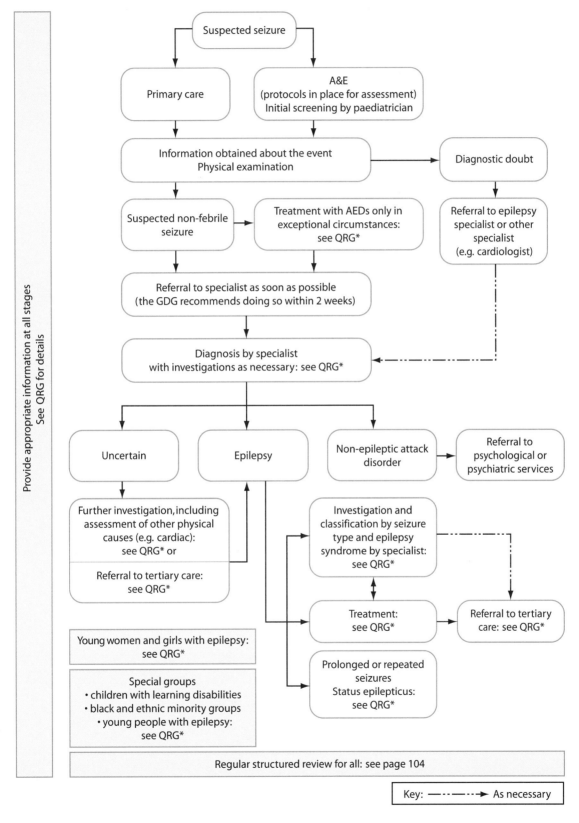

Differential diagnosis of epilepsy in adults

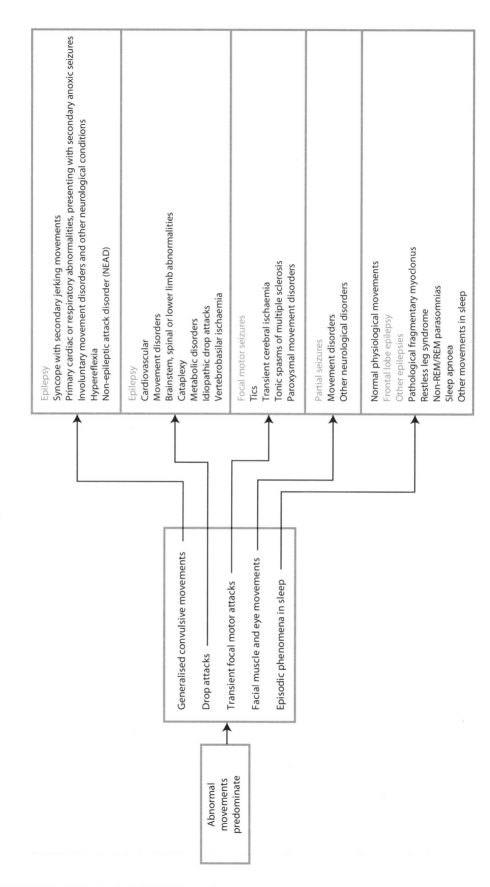

Abnormal movements predominate

- Generalised convulsive movements
- Drop attacks
- Transient focal motor attacks
- Facial muscle and eye movements
- Episodic phenomena in sleep

Epilepsy
Syncope with secondary jerking movements
Primary cardiac or respiratory abnormalities, presenting with secondary anoxic seizures
Involuntary movement disorders and other neurological conditions
Hyperreflexia
Non-epileptic attack disorder (NEAD)

Epilepsy
Cardiovascular
Movement disorders
Brainstem, spinal or lower limb abnormalities
Cataplexy
Metabolic disorders
Idiopathic drop attacks
Vertebrobasilar ischaemia

Focal motor seizures
Tics
Transient cerebral ischaemia
Tonic spasms of multiple sclerosis
Paroxysmal movement disorders

Partial seizures
Movement disorders
Other neurological disorders

Normal physiological movements
Frontal lobe epilepsy
Other epilepsies
Pathological fragmentary myoclonus
Restless leg syndrome
Non-REM/REM parasomnias
Sleep apnoea
Other movements in sleep

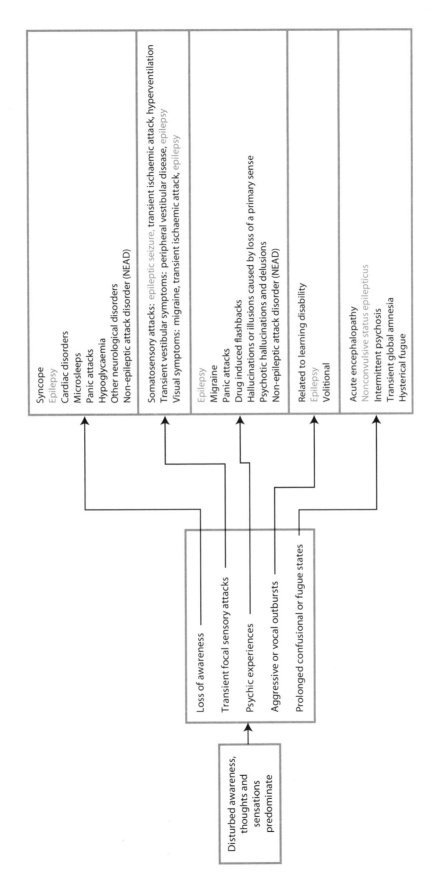

Disturbed awareness, thoughts and sensations predominate

Loss of awareness

Syncope
Epilepsy
Cardiac disorders
Microsleeps
Panic attacks
Hypoglycaemia
Other neurological disorders
Non-epileptic attack disorder (NEAD)

Transient focal sensory attacks

Somatosensory attacks: epileptic seizure, transient ischaemic attack, hyperventilation
Transient vestibular symptoms: peripheral vestibular disease, epilepsy
Visual symptoms: migraine, transient ischaemic attack, epilepsy

Psychic experiences

Epilepsy
Migraine
Panic attacks
Drug induced flashbacks
Hallucinations or illusions caused by loss of a primary sense
Psychotic hallucinations and delusions
Non-epileptic attack disorder (NEAD)

Aggressive or vocal outbursts

Related to learning disability
Epilepsy
Volitional

Prolonged confusional or fugue states

Acute encephalopathy
Nonconvulsive status epilepticus
Intermittent psychosis
Transient global amnesia
Hysterical fugue

Epilepsy: regular structured review

Regular structured review: adults

Provide regular structured review:
- usually by the GP or by the specialist, depending on the person with epilepsy's circumstances, epilepsy or preferences
- at least once a year; frequency will depend on person's epilepsy and preferences.

Refer to secondary or tertiary care if:
- epilepsy is inadequately controlled (in the view of the specialist or the person with epilepsy)
- there are specific medical or lifestyle issues (for example, pregnancy or drug cessation).

Regular structured review: children

Provide regular structured review:
- by a specialist
- at least once a year, but probably more frequently (every 3–12 months). Frequency will depend on child's epilepsy and preferences, and should be agreed with the child and their family and/or carers, as appropriate.

At the review: adults and children

Consider treatment:
- effectiveness
- tolerability
- side effects
- adherence.

Discuss the treatment plan and potential lifestyle issues.

Ensure access to:
- information (see QRG)
- counselling services
- epilepsy specialist nurses
- timely and appropriate investigations
- referral to tertiary care (including surgery) where appropriate.

Epilepsy references

These guidelines are extracts from:

National Institute for Health and Clinical Excellence. *The Epilepsies: the diagnosis and management of the epilepsies in adults and children in primary and secondary care: NICE guideline 20*. London: NICE; 2004. Available at: www.nice.org.uk/nicemedia/pdf/CG020NICEguideline.pdf

Reproduced with permission.

Adams SM, Knowles PD. Evaluation of a first seizure. *Am Fam Physician.* 2007; **75**(9): 1342–7.

Cohen AF, Land GS, Breimer DD, *et al.* Lamotrigine, a new anticonvulsant: pharmacokinetics in normal humans. *Clin Pharmacol Ther.* 1987; **42**(5): 535–41.

Fitzpatrick AP, Cooper P. Diagnosis and management of patients with blackouts. *Heart.* 2006; **92**(4): 559–68.

Friedman MJ, Sharieff GQ. Seizures in children. *Pediatr Clin North Am.* 2006; **53**(2): 257–77.

Mattson RH, Cramer JA, Collins JF. A comparison of valproate with carbamazepine for the treatment of complex partial seizures and secondarily generalized tonic-clonic seizures in adults. *N Engl J Med.* 1992; **327**(11): 765–71.

Sadleir LG, Scheffer IE. Febrile seizures. *BMJ.* 2007; **334**(7588): 307–11.

Scottish Intercollegiate Guidelines Network. *Diagnosis and Management of Epilepsy in Adults: SIGN guideline 70*. Edinburgh: SIGN; 2003. Available at: www.sign.ac.uk/pdf/qrg70.pdf

Sirven JI, Fife TD, Wingerchuk DM, *et al.* Second-generation antiepileptic drugs' impact on balance: a meta-analysis. *Mayo Clin Proc.* 2007; **82**(1): 40–7.

Stokes T, Shaw EJ, Juarez-Garcia A, *et al. Clinical Guidelines and Evidence Review for the Epilepsies: diagnosis and management in adults and children in primary and secondary care*. London: Royal College of General Practitioners; 2004. Available at: www.nice.org.uk/nicemedia/pdf/CG020fullguideline.pdf

Wiebe S, Blume WT, Girvin JP, *et al.* A randomized, controlled trial of surgery for temporal-lobe epilepsy. *N Engl J Med.* 2001; **345**(5): 311–18.

12

GROWTH CHARTS

Figure 12.1 Birth to 36 months: Girls
Length-for-age and Weight-for-age percentiles

NAME _____

RECORD # _____

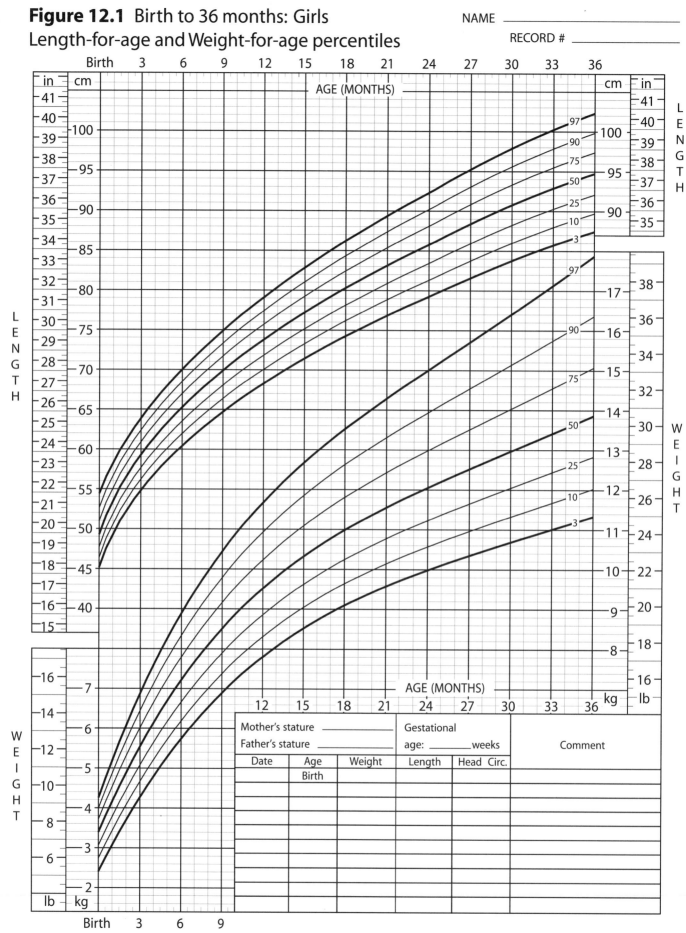

Published 30 May, 2000 (modified 20 April 2001).
SOURCE: Developed by the National Center for Health Statistics in collaboration with
the National Center for Chronic Disease Prevention and Health Promotion,
www.cdc.gov/growthcharts

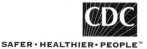

SAFER · HEALTHIER · PEOPLE™

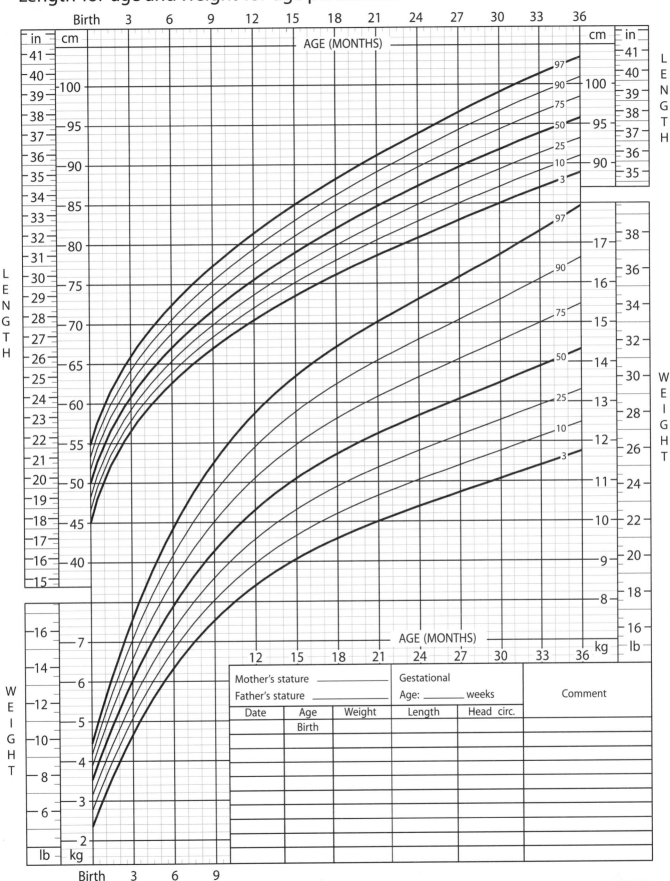

Figure 12.2 Birth to 36 months: Boys
Length-for-age and Weight-for-age percentiles

NAME _____

RECORD # _____

Published 30 May 2000 (modified 20 April 2001).
SOURCE: Developed by the National Center for Health Statistics in collaboration with
the National Center for Chronic Disease Prevention and Health Promotion,
www.cdc.gov/growthcharts

SAFER · HEALTHIER · PEOPLE™

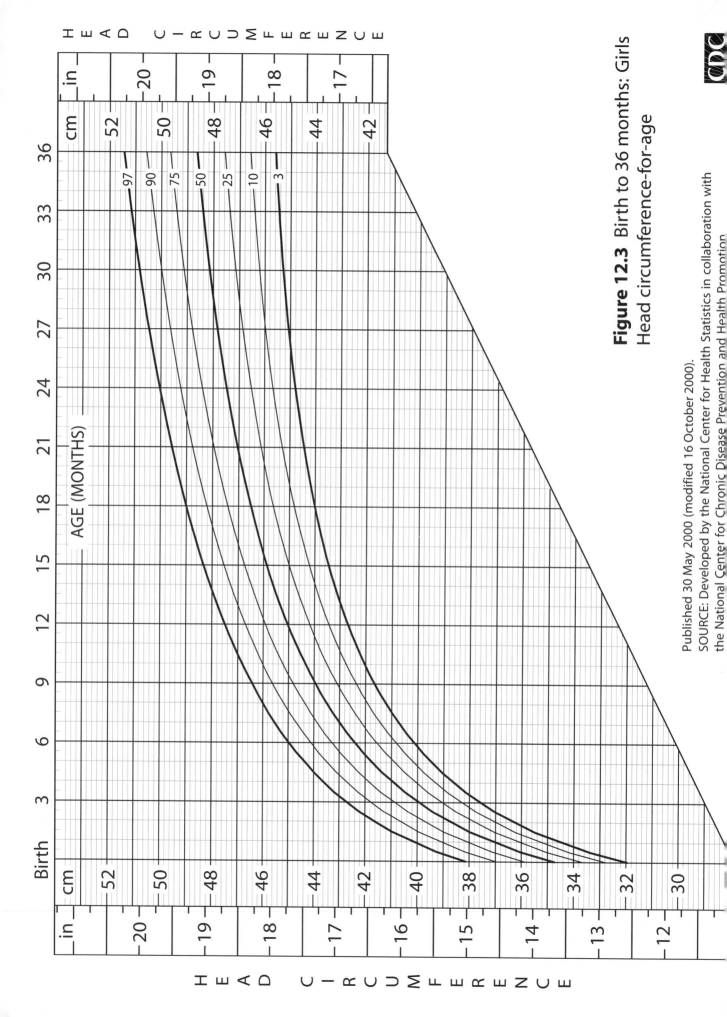

Figure 12.3 Birth to 36 months: Girls
Head circumference-for-age

Published 30 May 2000 (modified 16 October 2000).
SOURCE: Developed by the National Center for Health Statistics in collaboration with
the National Center for Chronic Disease Prevention and Health Promotion

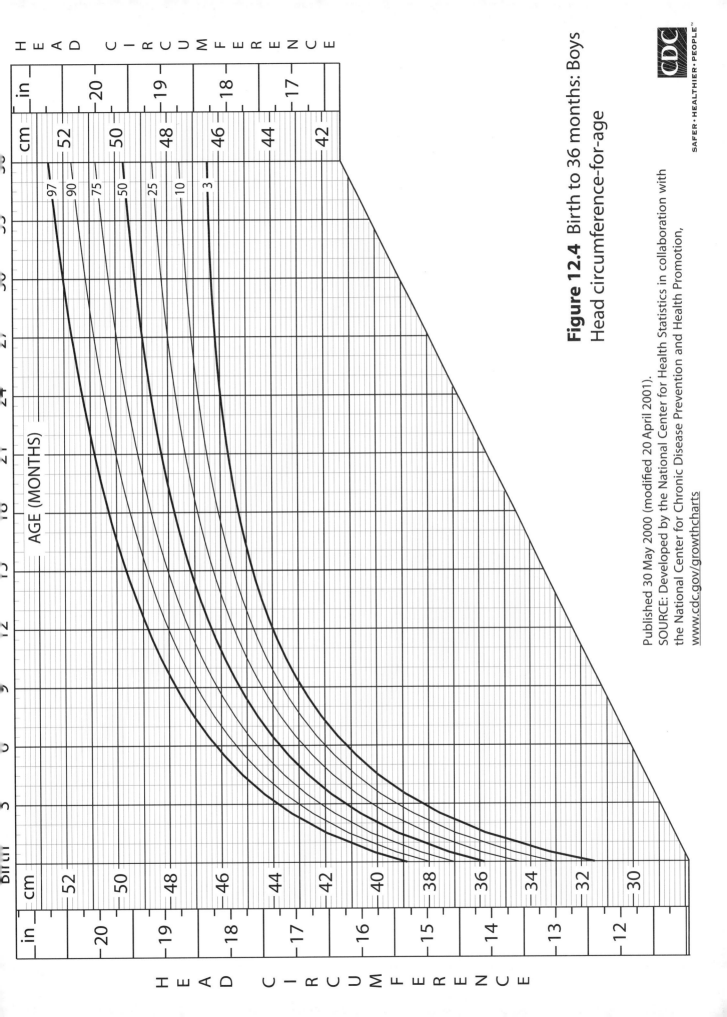

Figure 12.4 Birth to 36 months: Boys
Head circumference-for-age

Published 30 May 2000 (modified 20 April 2001).
SOURCE: Developed by the National Center for Health Statistics in collaboration with
the National Center for Chronic Disease Prevention and Health Promotion,
www.cdc.gov/growthcharts

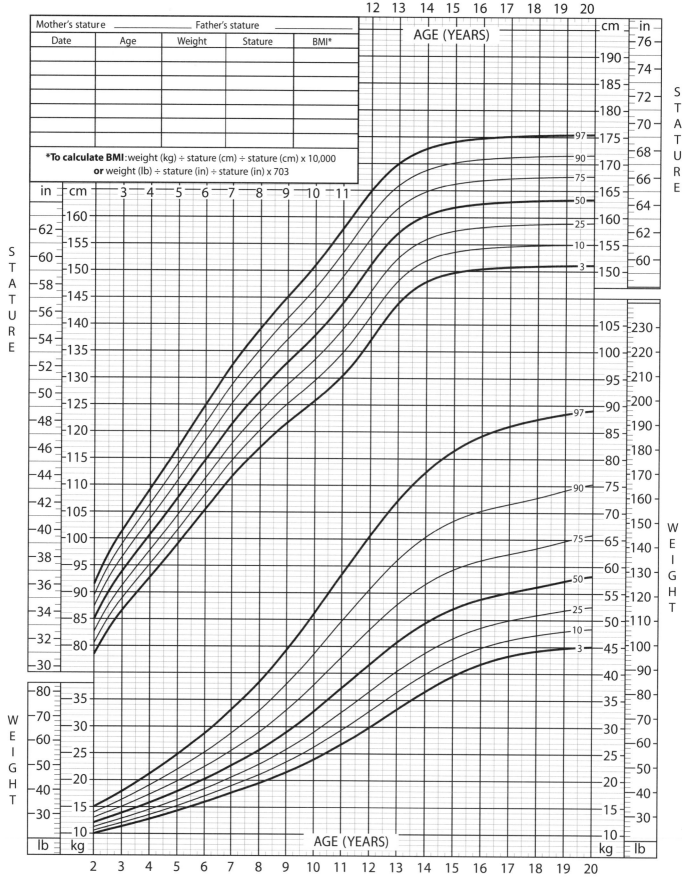

Figure 12.5 2 to 20 years: Girls
Stature-for-age and Weight-for-age percentiles

NAME _____

RECORD # _____

Mother's stature _____ Father's stature _____

Date	Age	Weight	Stature	BMI*

*To calculate BMI: weight (kg) ÷ stature (cm) ÷ stature (cm) x 10,000
or weight (lb) ÷ stature (in) ÷ stature (in) x 703

AGE (YEARS)

Published 30 May 2000 (modified 21 November 2000).
SOURCE: Developed by the National Center for Health Statistics in collaboration with
the National Center for Chronic Disease Prevention and Health Promotion,
www.cdc.gov/growthcharts

SAFER · HEALTHIER · PEOPLE™

Figure 12.6 2 to 20 years: Boys
Stature-for-age and Weight-for-age percentiles

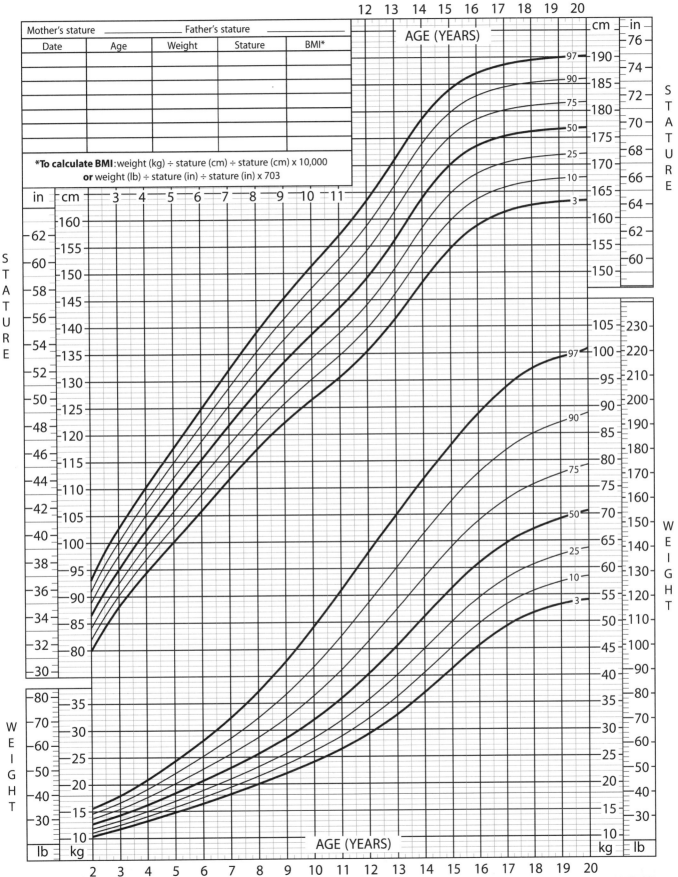

Published 30 May 2000 (modified 21 November 2000).
SOURCE: Developed by the National Center for Health Statistics in collaboration with
the National Center for Chronic Disease Prevention and Health Promotion,
www.cdc.gov/growthcharts

SAFER · HEALTHIER · PEOPLE™

Figure 12.7 2 to 20 years: Girls
Body mass index-for-age percentiles

NAME _____

RECORD # _____

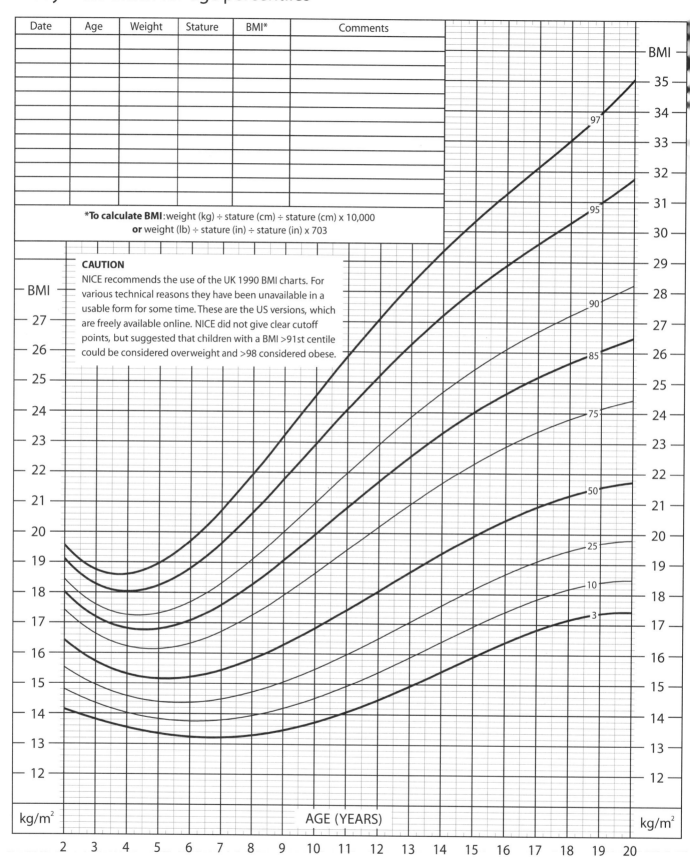

*To calculate BMI: weight (kg) ÷ stature (cm) ÷ stature (cm) x 10,000
or weight (lb) ÷ stature (in) ÷ stature (in) x 703

CAUTION
NICE recommends the use of the UK 1990 BMI charts. For various technical reasons they have been unavailable in a usable form for some time. These are the US versions, which are freely available online. NICE did not give clear cutoff points, but suggested that children with a BMI >91st centile could be considered overweight and >98 considered obese.

Published 30 May 2000 (modified 16 October 2000).
SOURCE: Developed by the National Center for Health Statistics in collaboration with the National Center for Chronic Disease Prevention and Health Promotion, www.cdc.gov/growthcharts

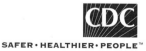

SAFER · HEALTHIER · PEOPLE™

Figure 12.8 2 to 20 years: Boys
Body mass index-for-age percentiles

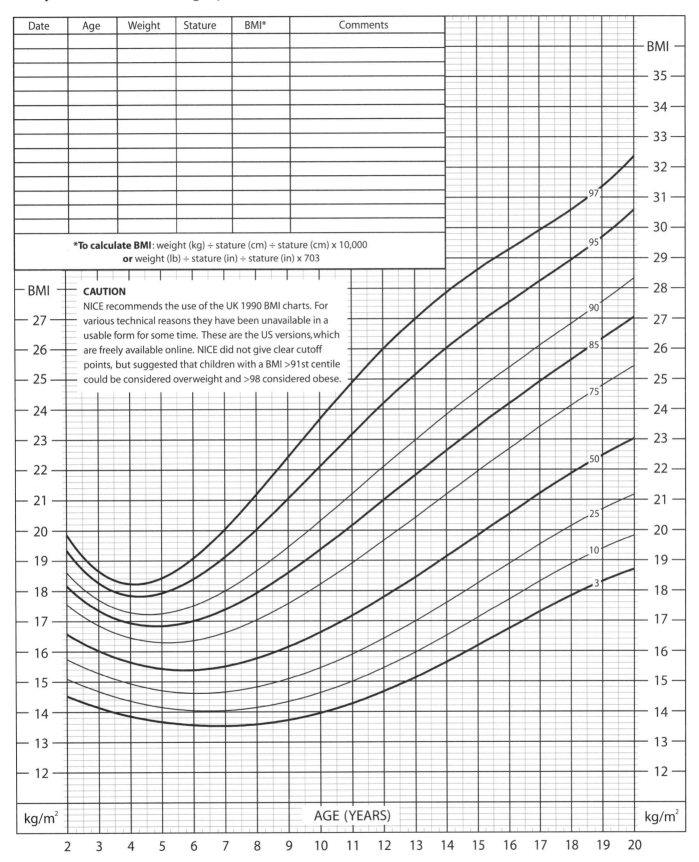

Date	Age	Weight	Stature	BMI*	Comments

*To calculate BMI: weight (kg) ÷ stature (cm) ÷ stature (cm) x 10,000
or weight (lb) ÷ stature (in) ÷ stature (in) x 703

CAUTION
NICE recommends the use of the UK 1990 BMI charts. For various technical reasons they have been unavailable in a usable form for some time. These are the US versions, which are freely available online. NICE did not give clear cutoff points, but suggested that children with a BMI >91st centile could be considered overweight and >98 considered obese.

AGE (YEARS)

Published 30 May 2000 (modified 16 October 2000).
SOURCE: Developed by the National Center for Health Statistics in collaboration with the National Center for Chronic Disease Prevention and Health Promotion, www.cdc.gov/growthcharts

CDC
SAFER · HEALTHIER · PEOPLE™

13

HEART FAILURE

Chronic heart failure 1

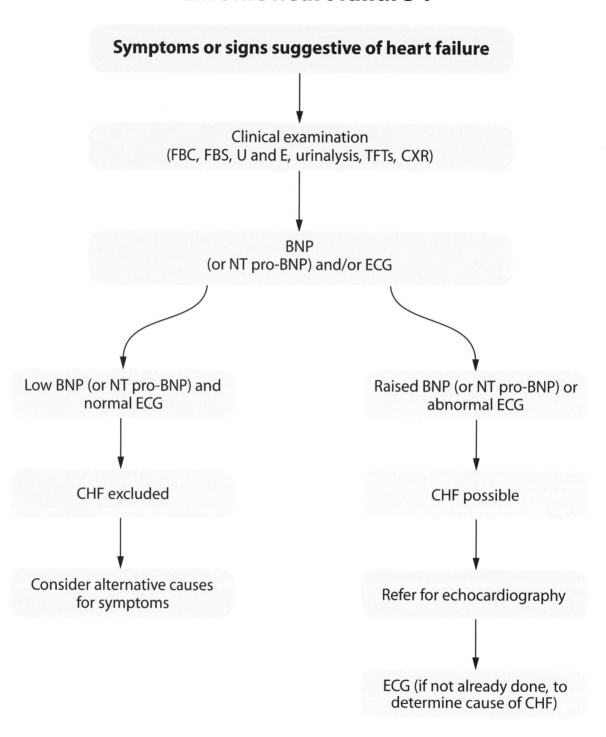

Symptoms or signs suggestive of heart failure

Clinical examination
(FBC, FBS, U and E, urinalysis, TFTs, CXR)

BNP
(or NT pro-BNP) and/or ECG

Low BNP (or NT pro-BNP) and normal ECG

CHF excluded

Consider alternative causes for symptoms

Raised BNP (or NT pro-BNP) or abnormal ECG

CHF possible

Refer for echocardiography

ECG (if not already done, to determine cause of CHF)

Chronic heart failure 2

Pharmacological therapies

ACE inhibitors

Ace inhibitors should be considered in patients with all NYHA functional classes of heart failure due to left ventricular systolic dysfunction

A

Beta blockers

All patients with heart failure due to LSVD of all NYHA functional classes should be started on beta blocker therapy as soon as their condition is stable (unless contraindicated by a history of asthma, heart block or symptomatic hypotension)

A

Angiotensin receptor blockers

Patients with chronic heart failure due to LSVD alone, or with heart failure, LVSD or both following myocardial infarction who are intolerant of ACE inhibitors should be considered for an angiotensin receptor blocker

A

Patients with HF due to LVSD who are still asymptomatic despite an ACE inhibitor and beta blocker may benefit from candesartan, following specialist advice

B

Aldosterone antagonists

Following specialist advice, patients with moderate to severe heart failure due to LVSD should be considered for spironolactone (unless contraindicated by renal impairment or high potassium)

B

Eplerenone can be substituted for spironolactone in patients who develop gynaecomastia

Patients who have had an MI with LV ejection fraction of ≤40% and diabetes or clinical signs of HF ahould be considered for epleronone (unless contraindicated by renal impairment or high potassium)

B

Diuretics

Should be considered for HF patients with dyspnoea or oedema (ankle or pulmonary)

B

Digoxin

Should be considered as an add-on therapy in HF patients in sinus rhythm who are still symptomatic after optimum therapy

B

NYHA functional classification in a patient with existing heart disease

Class I: No limitation during ordinary physical activity.
Class II: Slight limitation of physical activity. Develops fatigue or dyspnoea with moderate exercise.
Class III: Marked limitation of physical activity. Even light activity produces symptoms.
Class IV: Symptoms at rest. Any activity causes worsening.

Key: **A B C** Indicates grade of recommendation   Good practice point

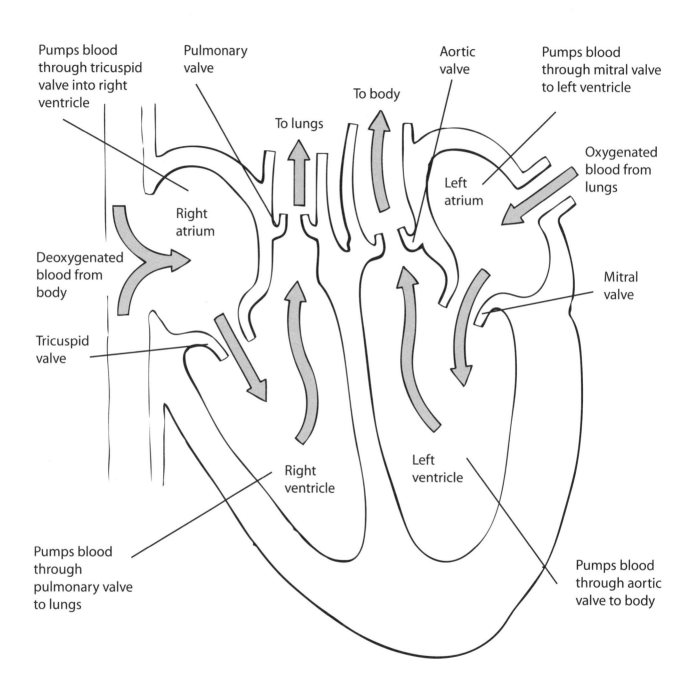

Figure 13.1 Blood flow through normal heart

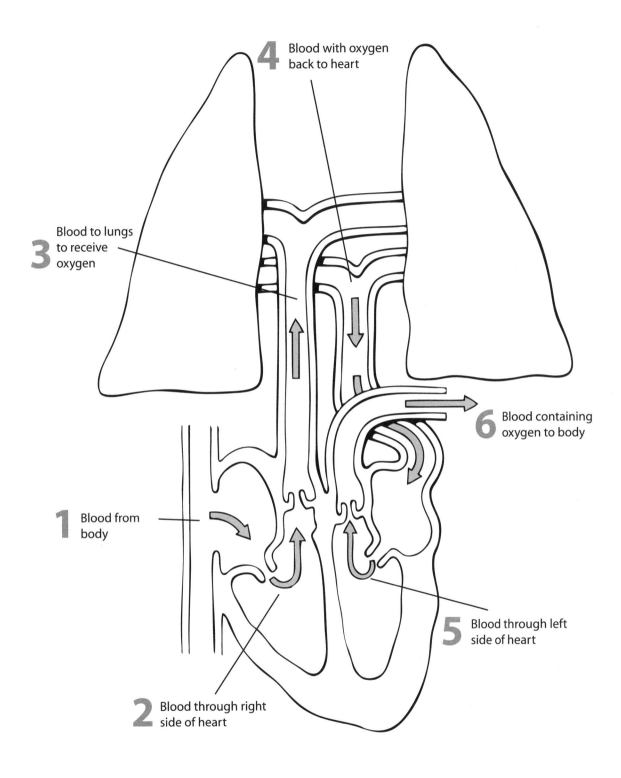

4 Blood with oxygen back to heart

3 Blood to lungs to receive oxygen

6 Blood containing oxygen to body

1 Blood from body

5 Blood through left side of heart

2 Blood through right side of heart

Figure 13.2 Blood flow through heart and lungs

Heart failure references

This guideline is an extract from:

Scottish Intercollegiate Guidelines Network. *The Management of Chronic Heart Failure: SIGN guideline 95*. Edinburgh: SIGN; 2007. Available at: www.sign.ac.uk/pdf/qrgchd.pdf

Dargie HJ, Lechat P. The Cardiac Insufficiency Bisoprolol Study II (CIBIS-II) beta blockers for mild to moderate heart failure. *Lancet*. 1999; **353**(9146): 9–13.

Digitalis Investigation Group. The effect of digoxin on mortality and morbidity in patients with heart failure. *N Engl J Med*. 1997; **336**(8): 525–33.

European Society of Cardiology. *Expert Consensus Document on Beta-Adrenergic Receptor Blockers*. Sophia Antipolis: ESC; 2004. Available at: www.escardio.org/guidelines-surveys/esc-guidelines/guidelinesdocuments/guidelines-bb-ft.pdf

European Society of Cardiology. *Guidelines on the Diagnosis and Treatment of Chronic Heart Failure*. Sophia Antipolis: ESC; 2005. Available at: www.escardio.org/guidelines-surveys/products/pocket/Pages/CHF.aspx

Flather MD, Yusuf S, Kober L, *et al*. Long-term ACE-inhibitor therapy in patients with heart failure or left-ventricular dysfunction: a systematic overview of data from individual patients. *Lancet*. 2000; **355**(9215): 1575–81.

Ghio S, Magrini G, Serio A, *et al*. on behalf of the SENIORS investigators. Effects of nebivolol in elderly heart failure patients with or without systolic left ventricular dysfunction: results of the SENIORS echocardiographic substudy. *Eu Heart J*. 2006; **27**(5): 562–8.

MERIT-HF Study Group. Effect of metoprolol CR/XL in chronic heart failure: Metoprolol CR/XL Randomised Intervention Trial in Congestive Heart Failure (MERIT-HF). *Lancet*. 1999; **353**(9169): 2001–7.

National Institute for Health and Clinical Excellence. *Chronic Heart Failure: Management of Chronic Heart Failure in Adults in Primary and Secondary Care: NICE guideline 5*. London: NICE; 2003. Available at: www.nice.org.uk/Guidance/CG5

Pitt B, Zannad F, Remme WJ, *et al*. The effect of spironolactone on morbidity and mortality in patients with severe heart failure. *N Engl J Med*. 1999; **341**(10): 709–17.

Steven Z, Pantilat MD, Steimle A. Palliative care for patients with heart failure. *JAMA*. 2004; **291**(20): 2476–82.

14

HYPERTENSION

Care pathway for hypertension

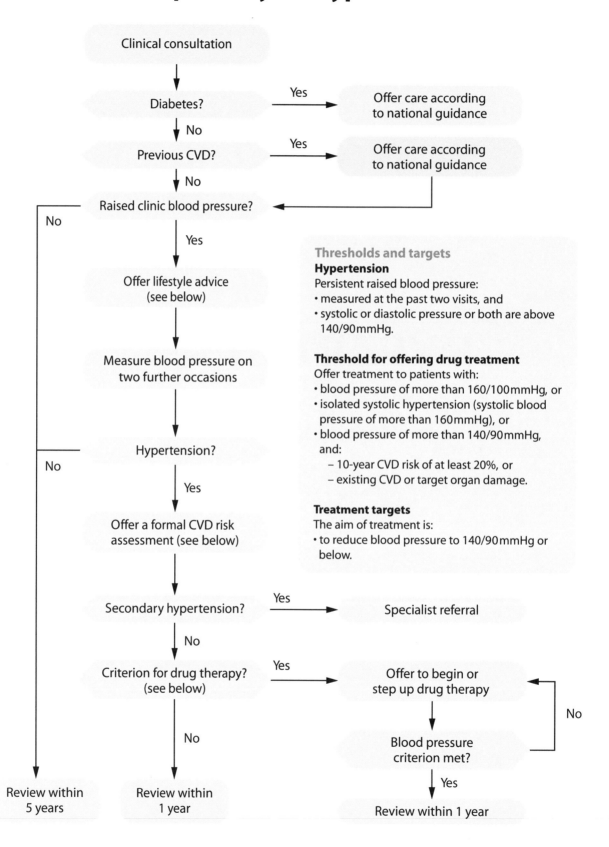

Clinical consultation

Diabetes? — Yes → Offer care according to national guidance

No

Previous CVD? — Yes → Offer care according to national guidance

No

Raised clinic blood pressure?

No (left branch)

Yes

Offer lifestyle advice (see below)

Measure blood pressure on two further occasions

Hypertension?

No (left branch)

Yes

Offer a formal CVD risk assessment (see below)

Secondary hypertension? — Yes → Specialist referral

No

Criterion for drug therapy? (see below) — Yes → **Offer to begin or step up drug therapy**

No

Blood pressure criterion met? — No (loop back to Offer to begin or step up drug therapy)

Yes → Review within 1 year

Review within 5 years

Review within 1 year

Thresholds and targets
Hypertension
Persistent raised blood pressure:
- measured at the past two visits, and
- systolic or diastolic pressure or both are above 140/90 mmHg.

Threshold for offering drug treatment
Offer treatment to patients with:
- blood pressure of more than 160/100 mmHg, or
- isolated systolic hypertension (systolic blood pressure of more than 160 mmHg), or
- blood pressure of more than 140/90 mmHg, and:
  – 10-year CVD risk of at least 20%, or
  – existing CVD or target organ damage.

Treatment targets
The aim of treatment is:
- to reduce blood pressure to 140/90 mmHg or below.

Hypertension – general management

Cardiovascular risk

- If raised blood pressure persists and the patient does not have established cardiovascular disease, discuss the need to formally assess their cardiovascular risk.
- Use the cardiovascular risk assessment to discuss prognosis and options for managing both raised blood pressure and other modifiable risk factors.
- Consider whether specialist referral is needed (see below).

Tests to assess risk
- Urine test for protein (using test strip).
- Plasma glucose, electrolytes, creatinine, serum total cholesterol and HDL cholesterol.
- 12-lead electrocardiography.

Lifestyle interventions to reduce blood pressure

- Ask patients about their diet and exercise patterns, and offer guidance and written or audiovisual information.
- Ask about alcohol consumption, and encourage patients to cut down if they drink excessively.
- Discourage excessive consumption of coffee and other caffeine-rich products.
- Encourage patients to reduce their salt intake or use a substitute.
- Offer smokers advice and help to stop smoking.
- Tell patients about local initiatives (for example, those run by healthcare teams or patient organisations) that provide support and promote lifestyle change.

Not recommended
- Do not offer calcium, magnesium or potassium supplements to reduce blood pressure.
- Relaxation therapies can reduce blood pressure and patients may wish to try them. However, primary care teams are not recommended to provide them routinely.

When to refer

- Refer immediately if the patient has signs of:
  - accelerated (malignant) hypertension (blood pressure more than 180/110 mmHg with signs of papilloedema and/or retinal haemorrhage)
  - suspected phaeochromocytoma (possible signs include labile or postural hypotension, headache, palpitations, pallor and diaphoresis).

- Consider referral if:
  - the patient has unusual signs and symptoms
  - the patient has signs or symptoms suggesting a secondary cause
  - the patient's management depends critically on the accurate estimation of their blood pressure
  - the patient has symptoms of postural hypotension, or a fall in systolic blood pressure when standing of 20mmHg or more.

Choosing drugs for patients newly diagnosed with hypertension

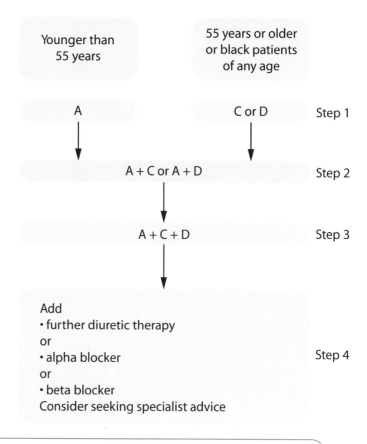

Abbreviations:
A = ACE inhibitor
(consider angiotensin-II receptor antagonist if ACE-intolerant)
C = calcium channel blocker
D = thiazide-type diuretic

Black patients are those of African or Caribbean descent; this does not include mixed race, Asian or Chinese patients

Younger than 55 years	55 years or older or black patients of any age	
A	C or D	Step 1
A + C or A + D		Step 2
A + C + D		Step 3

Add
• further diuretic therapy
or
• alpha blocker
or
• beta blocker
Consider seeking specialist advice   Step 4

Beta blockers
• Beta blockers are no longer preferred as a routine initial therapy for hypertension. But consider them for younger people, particularly:
  – women of childbearing potential
  – patients with evidence of increased sympathetic drive
  – patients with intolerance of or contraindications to ACE inhibitors and angiotensin-II receptor antagonists.

• If a patient taking a beta blocker needs a second drug, add a calcium-channel blocker rather than a thiazide-type diuretic, to reduce the patient's risk of developing diabetes.

• If a patient's blood pressure is not controlled by a regimen that includes a beta blocker (that is, it is still above 140/90 mmHg), change their treatment by following the flow chart above.

• If a patient's blood pressure is well controlled (that is, 140/90 mmHg or less) by a regimen that includes a beta blocker, consider long-term management at their routine review. There is no absolute need to replace the beta blocker in this case.

• When withdrawing a beta blocker, step down the dose gradually.

• Beta blockers should not usually be withdrawn if a patient has a compelling indication for being treated with one, such as symptomatic angina or a previous myocardial infarction.

BMI chart (adults)

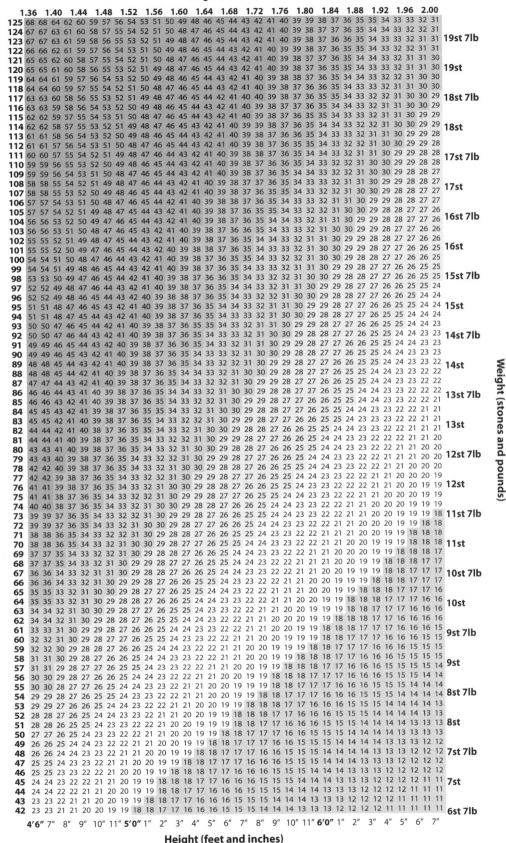

Figure 14.1 BMI chart (NICE and WHO definitions)

Hypertension references

This guideline is an extract from:

National Institute for Health and Clinical Excellence. *Management of Hypertension in Adults in Primary Care: NICE guideline 34* [partial update of NICE guideline 18]. London: NICE; 2006. Available at: www.nice.org.uk/CG34
Reproduced with permission.

ALLHAT Officers. Major outcomes in high-risk hypertensive patients randomized to angiotensin-converting enzyme inhibitor or calcium channel blocker vs diuretic. The Antihypertensive and Lipid-Lowering Treatment to Prevent Heart Attack Trial (ALLHAT). *J Am Med Assoc.* 2002; **288**(23): 2981–97.

Amery A, Birkenhager W, Brixko P, *et al.* Mortality and morbidity results from the European Working Party on High Blood Pressure in the Elderly Trial. *Lancet.* 1985; **1**(8442): 1349–54.

Carlberg B, Samuelsson O, Lindholm LH. Atenolol in hypertension: is it a wise choice? *Lancet.* 2004; **364**(9446): 1684–9.

Dahlof B, Hansson L, Lindholm L, *et al.* STOP hypertension morbidity and mortality in the Swedish Trial in Old Patients with Hypertension. *Lancet.* 1991; **338**: 1281–5.

Dahlöf B, Sever PS, Poulter NR, *et al.* Prevention of cardiovascular events with an antihypertensive regimen of amlodipine adding perindopril as required versus atenolol adding bendroflumethiazide as required, in the Anglo-Scandinavian Cardiac Outcomes Trial–Blood Pressure Lowering Arm (ASCOT–BPLA): a multicentre randomised controlled trial. *Lancet.* 2005; **366**(9489): 895–906.

Hansson L, Zanchetti I, Carruthers SG, *et al.* Effects of intensive blood-pressure lowering and low-dose aspirin in patients with hypertension: principal results of the Hypertension Optimal Treatment (HOT) Randomised Trial. *Lancet.* 1998; **351**(9118): 1755–62.

Hypertension Optimal Treatment Study Group. The Hypertension Optimal Treatment Study (The HOT Study). *Blood Pressure.* 1992; **2**: 62–8.

Joint British Societies. JBS 2: Joint British Societies' guidelines on prevention of cardiovascular disease in clinical practice. *Heart.* 2005; **91**(Suppl. 5): S1–52.

O'Brien E, Asmar R, Beilin L, *et al.* European Society of Hypertension recommendations for conventional, ambulatory and home blood pressure measurement. *J Hypertens.* 2003; **21**(5): 821–48.

Systolic Hypertension in the Elderly Program (SHEP) Cooperative Research Group. Prevention of stroke by antihypertensive drug treatment in older persons with isolated systolic hypertension. *JAMA.* 1991; **265**: 3255–64.

15

HYPOTHYROIDISM

Subclinical hypothyroidism
(not pregnant or planning a pregnancy)

What is subclinical hypothyroidism?

Subclinical hypothyroidism is diagnosed when there are no specific symptoms or signs of thyroid dysfunction but the thyroid-stimulating hormone (TSH) concentration is above the reference range and the free thyroxine (FT4) concentration is in the normal range, confirmed on repeat testing after at least 3 months.

How should I manage someone with subclinical hypothyroidism who has TSH <10 mU/L?

Levothyroxine treatment is not routinely recommended.
Consider levothyroxine treatment if there is a goitre or the TSH level is rising.
Consider a trial of levothyroxine treatment for people who have symptoms compatible with hypothyroidism.
• Prescribe treatment for a sufficient length of time to be able to judge whether there is symptomatic benefit.
• Only continue treatment if there is a clear improvement in symptoms.

If levothyroxine is not prescribed, measure serum thyroid peroxidase antibodies (TPO-Ab) and monitor thyroid function to detect progression to overt hypothyroidism.
• If the person has serum TPO-Ab, measure serum TSH annually or earlier if symptoms develop.
• If the person does not have serum TPO-Ab, measure serum TSH approximately every 3 years or earlier if symptoms develop.

How should I manage someone with subclinical hypothyroidism with TSH >10 mU/L?

If TSH concentration is greater than 10 mU/l and this finding is confirmed on repeated testing (at least 3 months later), many experts recommend treatment with levothyroxine.

How should levothyroxine be titrated?

Aim to achieve a serum TSH concentration that is within the reference range (0.4–4.5 mU/l).
In elderly people and people with a history of ischaemic heart disease, start with a low dose (consider levothyroxine 25 micrograms) and every 2–3 months titrate up by 25-microgram increments.
In younger people, start with levothyroxine 50–100 micrograms and every 2–3 months titrate up by 25- to 50-microgram increments.
Measure TSH and free thyroxine (FT4) 2–3 months after each change in dose of levothyroxine
Most people have a normal serum TSH concentration on a maintenance dose of 75–150 micrograms of levothyroxine daily.

How should I monitor someone who is stable on levothyroxine treatment?

Measure serum TSH at least once a year:
• to check compliance
• to ensure that the dosage is still correct.

When should I refer?

Seek specialist advice or refer people with hypothyroidism if any of the following apply:
• secondary hypothyroidism is suspected (refer urgently)
• subacute thyroiditis (de Quervain's thyroiditis) is suspected
• hypothyroidism is thought to be due to end-organ resistance
• they are younger than 16 years of age
• they are pregnant or postpartum
• they have particular management problems (e.g. ischaemic heart disease, or being treated with amiodarone or lithium)
• they feel worse during treatment, as they may have undiagnosed adrenal disease.

Overt hypothyroidism
(not pregnant or planning pregnancy)

What is overt hypothyroidism?

Overt hypothyroidism is caused by the undersecretion of thyroid hormone. It is diagnosed on the basis of characteristic clinical features and a serum thyroid-stimulating hormone (TSH) concentration greater than 10mU/l and a serum free thyroxine (FT4) concentration below the reference range.

How should I manage someone with overt hypothyroidism?

Treat overt hypothyroidism with levothyroxine.
All people who are stable on levothyroxine require at least annual measurement of serum TSH:
• to check compliance
• to ensure that the dosage is still correct.

How should levothyroxine be titrated?

Aim to achieve a serum TSH concentration that is within the reference range (0.4–4.5 mU/l).
In elderly people and people with a history of ischaemic heart disease, start with a low dose (consider levothyroxine 25 micrograms) and every 2–3 months titrate up by 25-microgram increments.
In younger people, start with levothyroxine 50–100 micrograms and every 2–3 months titrate up by 25- to 50-microgram increments.
Measure TSH and FT4 2–3 months after each change in dose of levothyroxine.
Most people have a normal serum TSH concentration on a maintenance dose of 75–150 micrograms of levothyroxine daily.

When should I refer?

Seek specialist advice or refer people with hypothyroidism if any of the following apply:
• secondary hypothyroidism is suspected (refer urgently)
• subacute thyroiditis (de Quervain's thyroiditis) is suspected
• hypothyroidism is thought to be due to end-organ resistance
• they are younger than 16 years of age
• they are pregnant or postpartum
• they have particular management problems (e.g. ischaemic heart disease, or being treated with amiodarone or lithium)
• they feel worse during treatment, as they may have undiagnosed adrenal disease.

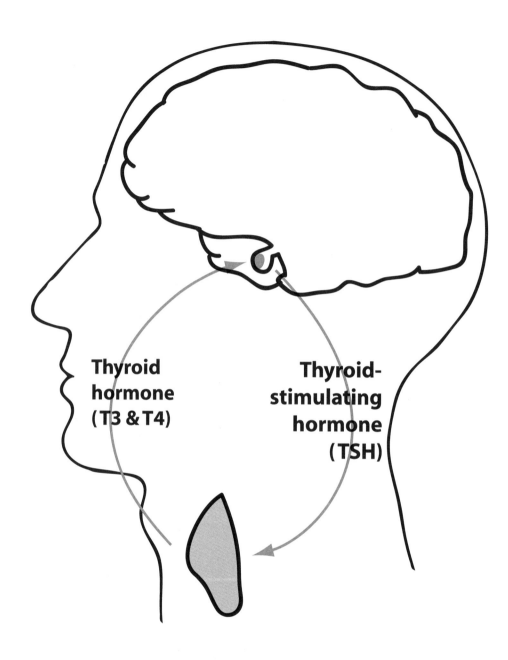

Figure 15.1 Simplified thyroid/pituitary negative feedback loop

Hypothyroidism references

These guidelines are an extract from the excellent online primary care resource Clinical Knowledge Summaries, www.cks.library.nhs.uk (the successor to PRODIGY).
Clinical Summary: Overt hypothyroidism. Available at: www.cks.library.nhs.uk/
hypothyroidism/management/quick_answers/scenario_subclinical_hypothyroidism
Clinical Summary: Subclinical hypothyroidism. Available at:
www.cks.library.nhs.uk/hypothyroidism/management/quick_answers/
scenario_overt_hypothyroidism
Reproduced with permission.

Association for Clinical Biochemistry, British Thyroid Association, British Thyroid Foundation. *UK Guidelines for the Use of Thyroid Function Tests.* ACB, BTA, BTF; 2006. Available at: www.british-thyroid-association.org/TFT_guideline_final_version_July_2006.pdf

Bandolier. Signs and symptoms predict thyroid disease. *Bandolier.* 1997. Available at: www.jr2.ox.ac.uk/bandolier/band46/b46-5.html#Heading3

Casey BM, Leveno KJ. Thyroid disease in pregnancy. *Obstet Gynecol.* 2006; **108**(5): 1283–92.

Cooper DS, Halpern R, Wood LC, *et al.* L-Thyroxine therapy in subclinical hypothyroidism: a double-blind, placebo-controlled trial. *Ann Intern Med.* 1984; **101**(1): 18–24.

Edwards A, Vanderpump M. *Hypothyroidism: diagnosis and treatment.* London: BMJ Learning; 2007. Available at: www.clinicalevidence.bmj.com/ceweb/besttreatments/abc/0605/0605_background.jsp?btuk=1#methods

Vanderpump M. Subclinical hypothyroidism: the case against treatment. *Trends Endocrinol Metab.* 2003; **14**(6): 262–6.

Vanderpump MPJ, Ahlquist JAO, Franklyn JA, *et al.* Consensus statement for good practice and audit measures in the management of hypothyroidism and hyperthyroidism. *BMJ.* 1996; **313**(7056): 539–44.

Walsh JP, Ward LC, Burke V, *et al.* Small changes in thyroxine dosage do not produce measurable changes in hypothyroid symptoms, well-being, or quality of life: results of a double-blind, randomized clinical trial. *J Clin Endocrinol Metab.* 2006; **91**(7): 2624–30.

Weetman AP. Hypothyroidism: screening and subclinical disease. *BMJ.* 1997; **314**(7088): 1175–8.

Wilson GR, Curry RW. Subclinical thyroid disease. *Am Fam Physician.* 2005; **72**(8): 1517–24.

16

INFERTILITY

Assessment and treatment for people with fertility problems

Initial advice for people concerned about delays in conception

- Cumulative probability of pregnancy in general population:
  - 84% in 1st year
  - 92% in 2nd year.
- Fertility declines with a woman's age.
- Lifestyle advice:
  - sexual intercourse every 2–3 days
  - ≤1–2 units alcohol/week for women; ≤3–4 units/week for men
  - smoking cessation programme for smokers
  - body mass index of 19–29
  - information about prescribed, over-the-counter and recreational drugs
  - information about occupational hazards.
- Offer preconceptional advice:
  - folic acid
  - rubella susceptibility and cervical screening.

Infertility:

failure to conceive after regular unprotected sexual intercourse for 2 years in the absence of known reproductive pathology.
This guideline does not include the management of people who are outside this definition, such as those with sexual dysfunction, couples who are using contraception and couples outside the reproductive age range.

Early investigation if:

history of predisposing factors (such as amenorrhoea, oligomenorrhoea, pelvic inflammatory disease or undescended testes); woman's age ≥35 yrs; people with HIV, hepatitis B and hepatitis C; prior treatment for cancer.

People preparing for cancer treatment

- Follow Royal College of Physicians and Royal College of Radiologists guidance.
- Cryostorage of gametes and/or embryos.

Principles of care

- Couple-centred management.
- Access to evidence-based information (verbal and written).
- Counselling from someone not directly involved in management of the couple's fertility problems.
- Contact with fertility support groups.
- Specialist teams.

Clinical investigation of fertility problems and management strategies
For people who have not conceived after 1 year of regular unprotected sexual intercourse

Female

Assessment of ovulation
Check for frequency and regularity of menstrual cycles.
If irregular:
✓ day 21 serum progesterone if 28 day cycle or later in long cycle to confirm ovulation
✓ serum gonadotrophins (FSH and LH)
✗ serum prolactin unless galactorrhoea or pituitary tumour
✗ inhibin B ✗ thyroid function test unless symptoms of thyroid disease ✗ endometrial biopsy.

Irregular ovulation   If regular ovulation, see
                       Unexplained infertility

WHO group I (hypothalamic pituitary failure)
⇨ Gonadotrophins with LH activity or pulsatile GnRH.
WHO group II (hypothalamic pituitary dysfunction, mainly polycystic ovary syndrome)
⇨ Clomifene citrate* or tamoxifen* (up to 12 months if ovulating) with ultrasound monitoring during at least the first cycle to adjust dose.
If ovulating but not pregnant after 6 months
⇨ Offer clomifene citrate* plus intra-uterine insemination.
If no ovulation with clomifene citrate
⇨ Metformin plus clomifene citrate* or
⇨ hMG*, uFSH* or rFSH* with ultrasound monitoring or
⇨ Ovarian drilling.
Hyperprolactinaemia:
⇨ Bromocriptine.   * Risk of OHSS and multiple pregnancy

Tests for tubal occlusion
The results of semen analysis and assessment of ovulation should be known before a test for tubal patency is performed.
✓ screening for Chlamydia trachomatis before uterine examination or offer prophylactic antibiotics.
✓ HSG/hysterosalpingo-contrast-ultrasonography if no history of co-morbidity (endometriosis/pelvic inflammatory disease/ectopic pregnancy).
✓ laparoscopy and dye if history of co-morbidity.

If occlusion   If normal

Consider in vitro fertilisation
⇨ Tubal surgery if mild tubal disease.
⇨ Tubal catheterisation or cannulation if proximal occlusion.
Minimal/mild endometriosis
⇨ Surgical ablation or resection and adhesiolysis at laparoscopy.
If no pregnancy
⇨ Stimulated intra-uterine insemination × 6 cycles with ultrasound monitoring with risk of OHSS and multiple pregnancy.
Moderate/severe endometriosis
⇨ Surgery.
Endometriomas
⇨ Laparoscopic cystectomy.

Unexplained fertility problems
(Normal semen analysis, no ovulation disorders, no tubal occlusion)
⇨ Clomifene citrate.
⇨ Unstimulated intra-uterine insemination × 6 cycles.
⇨ Fallopian sperm perfusion.

Male

Semen analysis
Compare with WHO reference values.
- Volume ≥2.0ml.
- Liquefaction time within 60 minutes.
- pH ≥7.2.
- Sperm concentration ≥20 × 10⁶ per ml.
- Total sperm number ≥40 × 10⁶ spermatozoa per ejaculate.
- Motility ≥50% (grades a and b) or ≥25% with progressive motility (grade a) within 60 minutes of ejaculation.
- Vitality ≥75% live.
- White blood cells: <10⁶ per ml.
- Morphology: 15% or 30%.
✗ Screening for anti-sperm antibodies.
✓ Ideally repeat after 3 months if abnormal or as soon as possible if gross sperm deficiency.

If abnormal   If normal, see Unexplained infertility

Hypogonadotrophic hypogonadism
⇨ Gonadotrophins.
Obstructive azoospermia
⇨ Surgery.
⇨ Sperm recovery.

Ejaculatory failure:
⇨ Drug therapy.
⇨ Sperm recovery.

Mild male factor fertility problems
⇨ Unstimulated intra-uterine insemination × 6 cycle.

Varicoceles
No surgery.

If no pregnancy with azoospermia, bilateral tubal occlusion or 3 years' infertility and the woman is aged 23–39 years, offer up to 3 stimulated cycles of in vitro fertilisation treatment

Procedures for in vitro fertilisation treatment

Additional principles of care for people undergoing in vitro fertilisation treatment

Access to evidence-based information (verbal and written) on risks/implications of assisted reproduction, including health of resulting children; genetic counselling; consideration of welfare of the child.

Factors affecting the outcome of in vitro fertilisation treatment

- Salpingectomy before in vitro fertilisation treatment for women with hydrosalpinges.
- Optimal woman's age is 23–39 years at time of treatment.
- Increased success with previous pregnancy and/or live birth.
- Ideal body mass index is 19–30.
- Increased success with low alcohol/caffeine intake.
- Increased success in non-smokers.
- Consistent for first 3 cycles of treatment, effectiveness after 3 cycles is uncertain.

1. Offer screening
✓ HIV, hepatitis B, hepatitis C; specialist referral if positive.

3. Embryo transfer
✓ No more than 2 embryos to be transferred during any 1 cycle.
✓ Offer cryostorage of supernumerary embryos if more than 2 embryos.
✓ Frozen embryos to be transferred before further stimulated cycles.
✓ Ultrasound-guided embryo transfer on day 2 or 3, or on day 5 or 6.

2. Ovulation induction
✗ Natural cycle.
✓ Pituitary down-regulation with GnRH agonist long protocol.
✓ GnRH agonist with gonadotrophins with consideration to minimising cost.
✗ GnRH antagonists.
✗ Growth hormone adjuvant.
✓ Monitor follicular development with ultrasound: clinics should have protocols for management of OHSS.
✓ Oocyte maturation with human chorionic gonadotrophins.
✗ Oocyte retrieval: offer conscious sedation (follow Academy of Medical Royal Colleges guidance).
✗ Follicle flushing.
✗ Assisted hatching.

4. Luteal support
✓ Progesterone.

Women should be informed of the risks of OHSS and multiple pregnancy

Management options associated with in vitro fertilisation treatment and other forms of assisted reproduction

Intracytoplasmic sperm injection – for couples with:
- severe semen quality deficits
- azoospermia
- poor in vitro fertilisation treatment response.

Screening
- Male karyotype.

Donor insemination – for couples with:
- azoospermia
- genetic/infectious disease in male partner
- severe rhesus isoimmunisation
- severe semen deficits.

Screening of sperm donors
- Follow British Andrology Society guidance
Assessment of female partner:
  - confirm ovulation
  - HSG if no pregnancy after 3 cycles.

Donor insemination – for women with
✓ Time insemination with either urinary luteinising hormone or basal body temperature changes.
✓ If regular ovulation, offer 6 unstimulated cycles.

Oocyte donation – for women with
- premature ovarian failure
- gonadal dysgenesis including Turner syndrome
- bilateral oophorectomy
- ovarian failure following chemotherapy or radiotherapy
- certain cases of in vitro fertilisation treatment failure
- genetic disorder transmission to offspring

Screening of oocyte donors
- Follow Human Fertilisation and Embryology Authority guidance.

Oocyte donors:
- Risks of ovarian stimulation and oocyte collection.
Egg sharing: counselling.

This algorithm should, where necessary, be interpreted with reference to the full guideline

Key: FSH = follicle-stimulating hormone; GnRH = gonadotrophin-releasing hormone; HIV = human immunodeficiency virus; hMG = human menopausal gonadotrophin; HSG = hysterosalpingography; LH = luteinising hormone; OHSS = ovarian hyperstimulation syndrome; rFSH = recombinant FSH; uFSH = urinary FSH; WHO = World Health Organization

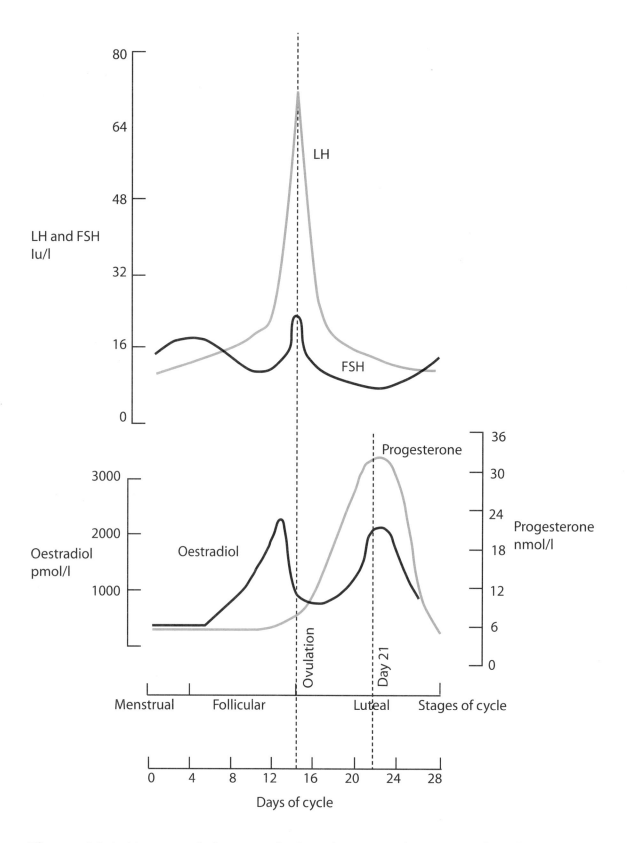

Figure 16.1 Hormonal changes during the normal menstrual cycle

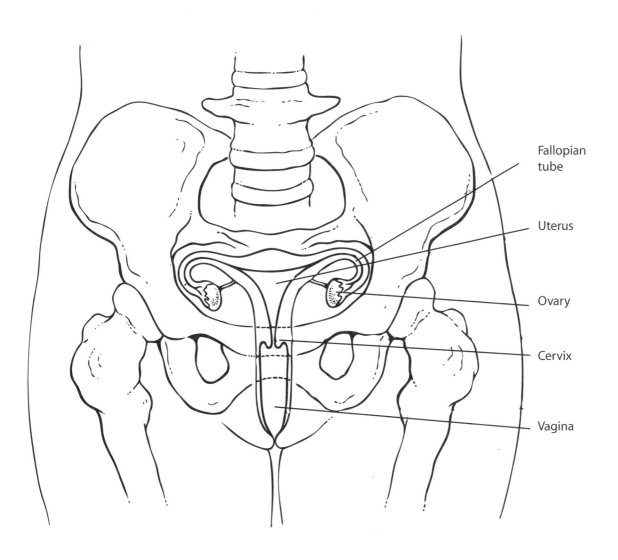

Fallopian tube

Uterus

Ovary

Cervix

Vagina

Figure 16.2 Female reproductive system in relation to pelvis

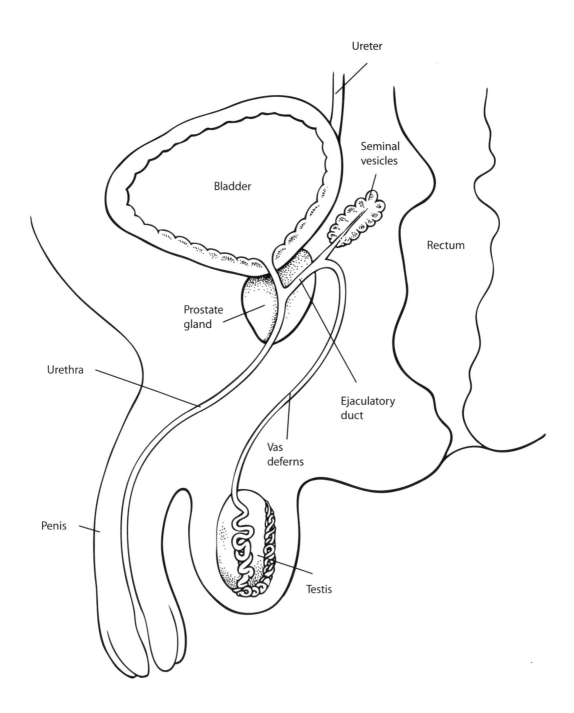

Figure 16.3 Normal male reproductive system

Infertility references

These guidelines are an extract from:

National Institute for Health and Clinical Excellence. *Assessment and Treatment for People with Fertility Problems: NICE guideline 11*. London: NICE; 2004. Available at: www.nice.org.uk/CG11

Reproduced with permission.

American Society for Reproductive Medicine. Current evaluation of amenorrhea. *Fertil Steril.* 2004; **82**(1): 266–72.

Braude P, Rowell P. Assisted conception: II. in vitro fertilisation and intracytoplasmic sperm injection [review]. *BMJ.* 2003; **327**(7419): 852–5.

British Fertility Society. *Risks and Complications of Assisted Conception.* Bradley Stoke: British Fertility Society; 2005. Available at: www.britishfertilitysociety. org.uk/public/factsheets/docs/BFS-risks%20and%20complications%20of%20 assisted%20conception%20.pdf

Cahill DJ, Wardel PG. Management of infertility. *BMJ.* 2002; **325**(7354): 28–32.

Cooke S. Treatment of infertility: the general approach to the infertile couple. *Prescr J.* 1996; **36**(1): 42–5.

Department of Health. *Updated Alcohol Advice for Pregnant Women.* London: DH; 2007. Available at: www.dh.gov.uk

Duckitt K. *Infertility and Subfertility.* London: BMJ Clinical Evidence; 2004.

Legro RS, Barnhart HX, Schlaff WD, *et al.* for the Cooperative Multicenter Reproductive Medicine Network. Clomiphene, metformin, or both for infertility in the polycystic ovary syndrome. *N Engl J Med.* 2007; **356**(6): 551–66.

Munkelwitz R, Gilbert BR. Are boxer shorts really better? A critical analysis of the role of underwear type in male subfertility. *J Urol.* 1998; **160**(4): 1329–33.

National Collaborating Centre for Women's and Children's Health. *Fertility: assessment and treatment for people with fertility problems.* London: Royal College of Obstetricians and Gynaecologists; 2004. Available at: www.rcog.org.uk/resources/ Public/pdf/Fertility_summary.pdf

17

OSTEOPOROSIS

Management of osteoporosis

Risk factors for osteoporosis

- Previous history of fracture.
- Female sex.
- Age >60 years.
- Family history of osteoporosis.
- Caucasian or Asian origin.

- Early menopause.
- Low body mass index (BMI=kg/m^2) .
- Smoking.
- Sedentary lifestyle.
- Long-term (≥3 months) corticosteroid use.

Diagnosis of osteoporosis

B	Conventional radiographs should not be used for the diagnosis or exclusion of osteoporosis	**B**	When plain films are interpreted as 'severe osteopoenia' it is appropriate to suggest referral for a DXA scan (dual-energy X-ray absorptiometry)
A	Bone mineral density (BMD) should normally be measured by DXA scanning performed on two sites, preferably AP spine and hip Repeat measurements should only be performed if they influence treatment	**C**	If DXA investigations are repeated, AP spine and total hip measurements should be used to follow response to treatment Following a DXA scan of the hip, the annual hip fracture risk (or 10-year fracture risk) should be included in the DXA report Where lateral spine scans acquired with fan-beam DXA are available, visual assessment should be used to assess prevalent vertebral fractures
A	Biochemical markers of bone turnover should have no role in the diagnosis of osteoporosis or in the selection of patients for BMD measurement		
B	Evidence of existing vertebral deformity should be used to modify the hip fracture risk estimated from age, sex and BMD		

Non-pharmacological management

A Post-menopausal women should aim for a dietary intake of 1000mg calcium per day

B
- High-intensity strength training is recommended as part of a management strategy for osteoporosis.
- Low-impact weight-bearing exercise is recommended as part of a management strategy for osteoporosis.
- Ipriflavone should not be used as a a sole therapy for fracture reduction in patients with osteoporosis.

Hormone replacement therapy (HRT)

☑ Use of HRT can be considered as a treatment option for osteoporosis, but the risks and benefit should be discussed with each individual woman before starting treatment

Bone mineral density (BMD)

The WHO working party stratified risk is as follows:

Normal
Bone mineral density less than 1 standard deviation below the young normal mean (T >-1)
Osteopaenia
Bone mineral density between 1 standard deviation and 2.5 standard deviations below the young normal mean (T between -1 and -2.5)
Osteoporosis
Bone mineral density more than 2.5 standard deviations below the young normal mean (T <-2.5)

This definition only applies to women

Key: **A B C D** Indicates grade of recommendation ☑ Good practice point

Osteoporosis – choosing drug therapy

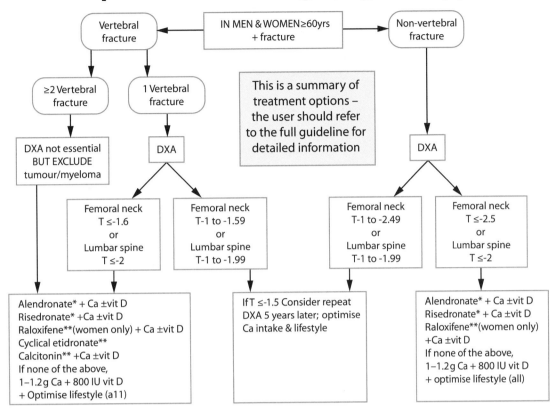

IN MEN & WOMEN≥60yrs + fracture

- Vertebral fracture
- Non-vertebral fracture

Vertebral fracture branch:

- ≥2 Vertebral fracture → DXA not essential BUT EXCLUDE tumour/myeloma
- 1 Vertebral fracture → DXA

This is a summary of treatment options – the user should refer to the full guideline for detailed information

≥2 Vertebral fracture / Femoral neck T ≤-1.6 or Lumbar spine T ≤-2:

Alendronate* + Ca ±vit D
Risedronate* +Ca ±vit D
Raloxifene**(women only) + Ca ±vit D
Cyclical etidronate**
Calcitonin** +Ca ±vit D
If none of the above,
1–1.2g Ca + 800 IU vit D
+ Optimise lifestyle (a11)

Femoral neck T-1 to -1.59 or Lumbar spine T-1 to -1.99:

If T ≤-1.5 Consider repeat DXA 5 years later; optimise Ca intake & lifestyle

Non-vertebral fracture → DXA:

Femoral neck T-1 to -2.49 or Lumbar spine T-1 to -1.99

Femoral neck T ≤-2.5 or Lumbar spine T ≤-2:

Alendronate* + Ca ±vit D
Risedronate* + Ca ±vit D
Raloxifene**(women only) +Ca ±vit D
If none of the above,
1–1.2g Ca + 800 IU vit D
+ optimise lifestyle (all)

*= Vertebral and non-vertebral fracture risk reduction ** = Reduction in vertebral fracture risk

Pharmacological management

In postmenopausal women with multiple vertebral fractures

- To reduce fracture risk at all sites, treat with oral risedronate (5mg daily or 35mg once weekly + calcium ± vitamin D).
- To reduce vertebral fracture risk, treat with intermittent cyclical etidronate (400mg daily for 14 days + 500mg calcium daily for 76 days, repeating 3-monthly cyclical therapy).

In postmenopausal women with osteoporosis determined by axial DXA and with a history of at least one vertebral fracture

- To reduce fracture risk at all sites, treat with oral alendronate (10mg daily or 70mg once weekly + calcium ± vitamin D).
- To reduce vertebral fracture risk, treat with oral raloxifene (60mg daily + calcium ± vitamin D).
- To reduce vertebral fracture risk, treat with intranasal calcitonin (200IU daily + calcium ± vitamin D).

In postmenopausal women with osteoporosis determined by axial DXA with or without previous non-vertebral fracture

- To reduce fracture risk at all sites, treat with either: oral alendronate (10mg daily or 70mg once weekly + calcium ± vitamin D) or oral risedronate (5mg daily or 35mg once weekly + calcium ± vitamin D).
- To reduce vertebral fracture risk, treat with oral raloxifene (60mg per day + calcium ± vitamin D).

In frail, elderly women (aged 80+ years) with a diagnosis of osteoporosis, with or without previous osteoporotic fractures

- To reduce fracture risk at all sites, elderly women who have suffered multiple vertebral fractures or who have had osteoporosis confirmed by DXA scanning should be considered for treatment with either oral risedronate (5mg daily or 35mg once weekly + calcium ± vitamin D) or oral alendronate (10mg daily or 70mg once weekly + calcium ± vitamin D).
- To reduce hip fracture risk, frail elderly women who are housebound should receive oral calcium (1000–1200mg daily + 800IU vitamin D).

In men with a diagnosis of osteoporosis, with or without previous osteoporotic fractures

- To reduce fracture risk at all sites, men with low BMD and/or history of one or more vertebral fractures or one non-vertebral steoporotic fracture should be treated with oral alendronate (10mg + 500mg calcium +/- 400IU vitamin D daily).

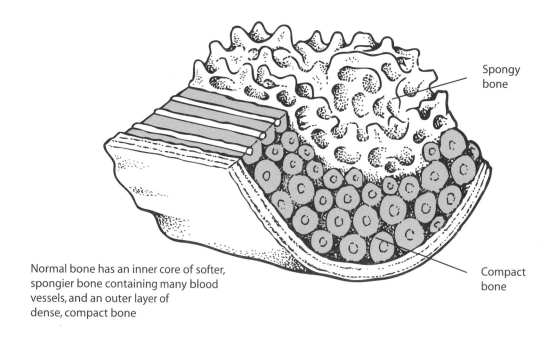

Spongy
bone

Compact
bone

Normal bone has an inner core of softer,
spongier bone containing many blood
vessels, and an outer layer of
dense, compact bone

Figure 17.1a Normal bone structure

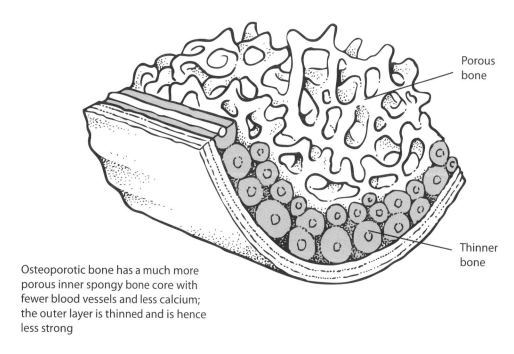

Porous
bone

Thinner
bone

Osteoporotic bone has a much more
porous inner spongy bone core with
fewer blood vessels and less calcium;
the outer layer is thinned and is hence
less strong

Figure 17.1b Osteoporotic bone

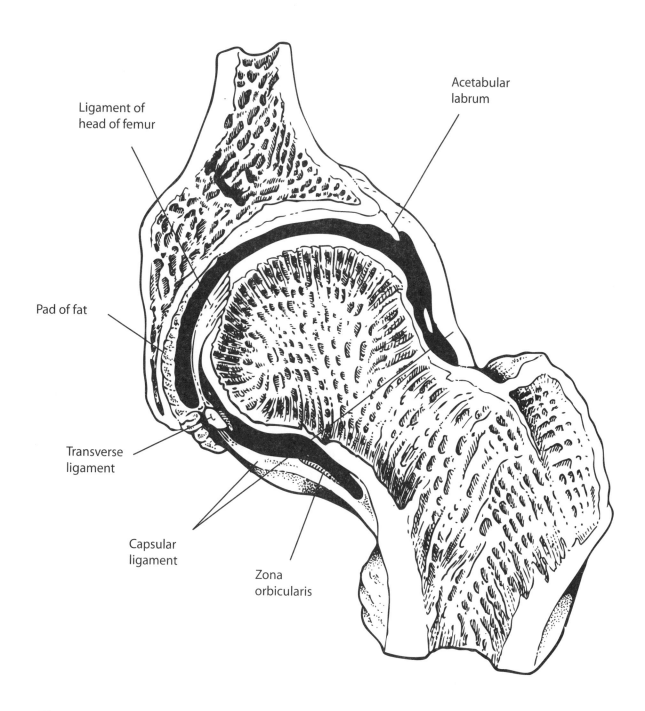

Figure 17.2 Normal hip joint

Osteoporosis references

This guideline is an extract from:
Scottish Intercollegiate Guidelines Network. *Management of Osteoporosis: SIGN guideline 71.* Edinburgh: SIGN; 2003. Available at: www.sign.ac.uk/pdf/ qrg71.pdf

Arlot ME, Delmas PD and Meunier PJ. Effect of calcium and cholecalciferol treatment for three years on hip fractures in elderly women. *BMJ.* 1994; **308**(6936), 1081–2.

Ascott-Evans BH, Guanabens N, Kivinen S, et al. Alendronate prevents loss of bone density associated with discontinuation of hormone replacement therapy: a randomized controlled trial. *Arch Intern Med.* 2003; **163**(7): 789–94.

Black DM, Cummings SR, Karpf DB, *et al.* Randomised trial of effect of alendronate on risk of fracture in women with existing vertebral fractures. *Lancet.* 1996; **348**(9041): 1535–41.

Cummings SRM, Palermo L, Browner W, *et al.* Monitoring osteoporosis therapy with bone densitometry: misleading changes and regression to the mean. *JAMA.* 2000; **283**(10): 1318–21.

Greenspan SL, Bone G, Schnitzer TJ, *et al.* Two-year results of once-weekly administration of alendronate 70 mg for the treatment of postmenopausal osteoporosis. *J Bone Miner Res.* 2002; **17**(11): 1988–96.

Kanis JA, Johnell O, De Laet C, *et al.* A meta-analysis of previous fracture and subsequent fracture risk. *Bone.* 2004; **35**(2): 375–82.

Khan AA, Hodsman AB, Papaioannou A, *et al.* Management of osteoporosis in men: an update and case example [review]. *CMAJ.* 2007; **176**(3): 345–8.

McClung MR, Geusens P, Miller PD, *et al.* Effect of risedronate on the risk of hip fracture in elderly women. *N Engl J Med.* 2001; **344**(5): 333–40.

Orwoll E, Ettinger M, Weiss S, *et al.* Alendronate for the treatment of osteoporosis in men. *N Engl J Med.* 2000; **343**(9): 604–10.

Poole KE, Compston JE. Osteoporosis and its management [review]. *BMJ.* 2006; **333**(7581): 1251–6.

Torgerson DJ, Bell-Syer SE. Hormone replacement therapy and prevention of nonvertebral fractures: a meta-analysis of randomized trials. *JAMA.* 2001; **285**(22): 2891–7.

18

OTITIS MEDIA

Otitis media

	Earache, fever, irritability	Middle ear effusion	Opaque drum	Bulging drum	Impaired drum mobility	Hearing loss
Diagnostic features of acute otitis media (AOM) & otitis media with effusion (OME, Glue Ear)						
AOM	Present	Present	Present	May be present	Present	Present
OME	Usually absent	Present	May be absent	Usually absent	Present	Usually present

Treatment

Acute otitis media

In the majority of cases, AOM is a self-limiting condition

Antibiotics

Children diagnosed with AOM should not be routinely prescribed antibiotics as the initial treatment **B**

If an antibiotic is to be prescribed, the conventional 5-day course is recommended at dosage levels indicated in the BNF **B**

Decongestants, antihistamines, mucolytics

Children with AOM should not be prescribed decongestants or antihistamines **A**

Analgesics

Parents should give paracetamol for analgesia but should be advised of the potential danger of overuse **D**

Oils

Insertion of oils should not be prescribed for reducing pain in children with AOM **B**

Homeopathy

Insufficient evidence to recommend in the management of AOM or OME

Referral for AOM

Children with frequent episodes (more than 4 in 6 months) of AOM, or with complications, should be referred to an otolaryngologist **D**

Otitis media with effusion

In the majority of cases, OME is a self-limiting condition

Antibiotics

Children diagnosed with otitis media with effusion should not be treated with antibiotics **D**

Decongestants, antihistamines, mucolytics

Decongestants, antihistamines, mucolytics should not be used in the management of OME **B**

Steroids

The use of either topical or systemic steroids is not recommended in the management of children with OME **B**

Autoinflation

May be of benefit in the management of some children with OME **D**

Referral for OME

Children under 3 with persistent OME and hearing loss ≤25dB, but no speech and language, developmental or behavioural problems, can be safely managed with watchful waiting. If watchful waiting is being considered, the child should undergo audiometry to exclude a more serious degree of hearing loss **A**

Children with persistent bilateral OME over 3 years of age or who have speech and language, developmental or behavioural problems should be referred to an otolaryngologist **B**

Key: **A B C D** Indicates grade of recommendation

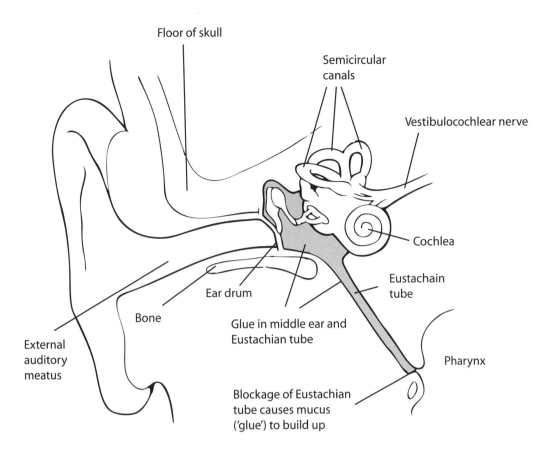

Figure 18.1a Glue ear

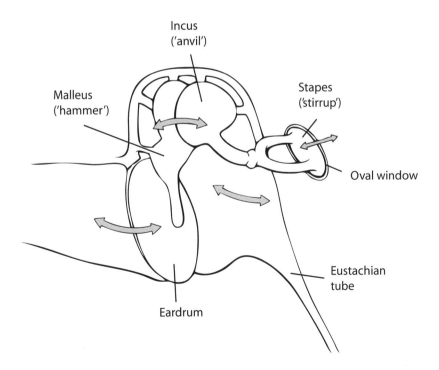

Figure 18.1b Movement of ossicles

Otitis media references

These guidelines are an extract from:

Scottish Intercollegiate Guidelines Network. *Diagnosis and Management of Childhood Otitis Media in Primary Care: SIGN guideline 66.* Edinburgh: SIGN; 2003. Available at: www.sign.ac.uk/pdf/qrg66.pdf

American Academy of Pediatrics. Diagnosis and management of acute otitis media. *Pediatrics.* 2004; **113**(5): 1451–65.

Arrieta A, Singh J. Management of recurrent and persistent acute otitis media: new options with familiar antibiotics. *Pediatr Infect Dis J.* 2004; **23**(Suppl. 2): S115–24.

Arroll B, Kenealy T, Kerse N. Do delayed prescriptions reduce antibiotic use in respiratory tract infections? A systematic review. *Br J Gen Pract.* 2003; **53**(496): 871–7.

Cates C. An evidence-based approach to reducing antibiotic use in children with acute otitis media: controlled before and after study. *BMJ.* 1999; **318**(7185): 715.

Damoiseaux RA, Rovers MM, van Balen FA, *et al.* Long-term prognosis of acute otitis media in infancy: determinants of recurrent acute otitis media and persistent middle ear effusion. *Fam Pract.* 2006: **23**(1): 40–5.

Little P, Moore M, Warner G, *et al.* Longer-term outcomes from a randomised trial of prescribing strategies in otitis media. *Br J Gen Pract.* 2006; **56**(524): 176–82.

McCormick DP, Chonmaitree T, Pittman C, *et al.* Non-severe acute otitis media: a clinical trial comparing outcomes of watchful waiting versus immediate antibiotic treatment *Pediatrics.* 2005; **115**(6): 1455–65.

Rimmer J, Giddings CE, Weir N. History of myringotomy and grommets. *J Laryngol Otol.* 2007; **121**(10): 911–16.

Rovers MM, Glasziou P, Appelman CL, *et al.* Antibiotics for acute otitis media: a meta-analysis with individual patient data. *Lancet.* 2006; **368**(9545): 1429–35.

Spiro DM, Tay KY, Arnold DH, *et al.* Wait-and-see prescription for the treatment of acute otitis media: a randomized controlled trial. *J Am Med Assoc.* 2006; **296**(10): 1235–41.

19

POST-MENOPAUSAL BLEEDING

Post-menopausal bleeding

The following two pages, taken from the Quick Reference Guide, provide a summary of the main recommendations in the SIGN guideline on investigation of post-menopausal bleeding.

Definition

The menopause is the permanent cessation of menstruation resulting from the loss of ovarian follicular activity. From a symptomatic perspective, post-menopausal bleeding describes the occurrence of vaginal bleeding following a woman's last menstrual cycle. For the purposes of this guideline, an episode of bleeding 12 months or more after the last period is accepted as post-menopausal bleeding.

PMB and HRT

C Older HRT regimens that utilise unopposed oestrogen increase the relative risk of endometrial carcinoma by around six times after five years of use. Progestogens are added to HRT regimens to prevent endometrial hyperplasia and cancer: their inclusion reduces the relative risk of endometrial cancer to around 1.5

Unscheduled bleeding is the term used for breakthrough bleeding occurring in women on cyclical HRT or any bleeding in women on tibolone (Livial) or continuous combined HRT, although it can take up to six months for amenorrhoea to develop in the latter treatments

For sequential regimens, abnormal bleeding may:
• be heavy or prolonged at the end of or after the progestogen phase, or
• occur at any time (breakthrough bleeding)

For continuous combined regimens, bleeding should be considered abnormal (requiring endometrial assessment) if:
• it occurs after the first six months of treatment, or
• it occurs after amenorrhoea has been established.

Clinicians should be aware of the background incidence of endometrial cancer among users and non-users of HRT and in those who present with post-menopausal bleeding

PMB and tamoxifen

A Women receiving tamoxifen in the treatment or prevention of breast cancer experience a 3- to 6-fold greater incidence of endometrial cancer

Clinicians should be aware that post-menopausal women receiving tamoxifen therapy, particularly for longer than 5 years, are at increased risk of endometrial cancer

Investigation of PMB

☑ In patients on sequential HRT, TVUS measurements should take place during the first half of the cycle where possible

D D&C should no longer be used as the primary method of investigating PMB

Hysteroscopy

B Outpatient techniques for hysteroscopy and suction sampling of the endometrium should be available in all diagnostic units

B Facilities to perform hysteroscopy and curettage under general anaesthetic should be available for when the outpatient procedure is not possible or the patient has a strong preference for a general anaesthetic

Endometrial biopsy

C Histological specimens may be obtained either at the same time as inpatient or outpatient hysteroscopy with curettage or by using an endometrium sampling device, e.g. Pipelle™

Recurrent PMB

☑ Re-investigation of recurrent post-menopausal bleeding should be considered after six months

---

Key: **A B C D** Indicates grade of evidence   ☑ Good practice point

ALL WOMEN WITH PMB	WOMEN USING HRT	WOMEN USING TAMOXIFEN

Referral

GPs should take into account patterns of bleeding, their relationship to the use of HRT and patient preferences when considering a referral. Concern from either general practitioner or patient about the possibility of PMB signalling endometrial cancer constitutes sufficient grounds for referral.

D The risk of endometrial cancer in non-HRT users complaining of PMB and in HRT users experiencing abnormal bleeding is sufficient to recommend referring patients for investigation

Women presenting with PMB require a pelvic examination at some stage during their assessment. If referred to a gynaecologist, an examination by the GP is not always necessary. However, examination by a GP or practice nurse can alter the course of clinical management if it expedites referral on grounds of raised suspicion of a malignancy.

Questions to ask in the assessment of patients with abnormal bleeding on HRT
- When does bleeding occur with respect to the oestrogen and the progestogen phase?
- How long does the bleeding last and how heavy is it?
- Was there a period of amenorrhoea before HRT was started?
- Is there a problem suggesting poor compliance?
- Is there a reason to suspect poor gastrointestinal absorption?
- Is the patient taking any other drugs?

Whether or not to continue HRT prior to investigation may depend on the patient's wishes and how long she has to wait. There is no specific reason for discontinuing HRT.

In view of the increased risk of endometrial cancer associated with tamoxifen therapy, there is a case for heightened vigilance for PMB by both the woman and the clinician(s) responsible for her care.

However, current evidence does not justify the use of any investigation (ultrasonography, hysteroscopy, endometrial biopsy or dilatation and curettage) in post-menopausal women receiving treatment with tamoxifen in the absence of vaginal bleeding.

Unnecessary investigation should be avoided as there are risks associated with further investigation.

C Endometrial investigation in post-menopausal women on tamoxifen should only be carried out in those experiencing vaginal bleeding.

Investigation

B Where sufficient local skills and capacity exist, transvaginal ultrasound is the first-line procedure* to identify which women with post-menopausal bleeding are at higher risk of endometrial cancer.

B An endometrial thickness of <3mm can be used to exclude endometrial cancer in women who:
- have never used HRT, OR
- have not used any form of HRT for >1 year, OR
- are using continuous combined HRT.

Estimated pre-test risk of cancer: 10%

≤3mm	>3mm
Post-test risk: 0.6–0.8%	20–22%

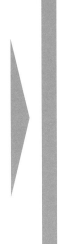

C Histological specimens may be obtained either at the same time as inpatient or outpatient hysteroscopy with curettage or using an endometrium sampling device, e.g. Pipelle™.

C Hysteroscopy and biopsy (curettage) is the preferred diagnostic technique to detect polyps and other benign lesions.

B If the clinician and the woman judge that the level of reassurance and reduced risk are acceptable following TVUS, no further action need be taken. Further investigations should be carried out if symptoms recur. If the clinician or patient are not satisfied with this level of reassurance, further investigation is justified. This should include an endometrial biopsy to obtain a histological assessment.

B An endometrial thickness of 5mm can be used to exclude endometrial cancer in women using sequential combined HRT (or having used it within the past year) with unscheduled bleeding.

Estimated pre-test risk: 1–1.5%

>5mm	≤5mm
Post-test risk: 2–5%	0.1–0.2%

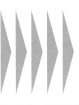

Ultrasonography is poor at differentiating potential cancer from other tamoxifen-induced thickening because of the distorted endometrial architecture associated with long-term use of tamoxifen.

D Hysteroscopy with biopsy is preferable as the first line of investigation in women taking tamoxifen who experience PMB.

Transabdominal ultrasound may be used as a complementary examination if the uterus is significantly enlarged or a wider view of the pelvis or abdomen is required. Transabdominal ultrasound may also be used in the small proportion of women in whom it proves technically impossible to perform a transvaginal ultrasound.

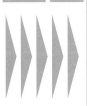

* The sequence of investigation will depend on clinical judgement, local resources and expertise, and patient preference. Obtaining an initial endometrial sample may be in the patient's interest if it identifies a cancer prior to the ultrasound appointment.

Postmenopausal bleeding references

This guideline is an extract from the SIGN quick reference guide:
Scottish Intercollegiate Guidelines Network. *The Investigation of Postmenopausal Bleeding: a national guideline: SIGN guideline 61*. Edinburgh: SIGN; 2002. Available at: www.sign.ac.uk/pdf/qrg61.pdf

Albers JR, Hull SK, Wesley RM. Abnormal uterine bleeding. *Am Fam Physician*. 2004; **69**(8): 1915–26.

Clark TJ, Voit D, Gupta JK, *et al*. Accuracy of hysteroscopy in the diagnosis of endometrial cancer and hyperplasia: a systematic quantitative review. *JAMA*. 2002; **288**(13): 1610–21.

Dijkhuizen FP, Mol BW, Brölmann HA, *et al*. The accuracy of endometrial sampling in the diagnosis of patients with endometrial carcinoma and hyperplasia: a meta-analysis. *Cancer*. 2000; **89**(8): 1765–72.

Greendale GA, Lee NP, Arriola ER. The menopause. *Lancet*. 1999; **353**(9152): 571–80.

Kerns JW, Mabry S, Lopez R. Clinical inquiries. What is the best diagnostic approach to postmenopausal vaginal bleeding in women taking hormone replacement therapy? *J Fam Pract*. 2001; **50**(10): 843–4.

Reinhold C, Khalili I. Postmenopausal bleeding: value of imaging. *Radiol Clin North Am*. 2002; **40**(3): 527–62.

Sahdev A. Imaging the endometrium in postmenopausal bleeding. *BMJ*. 2007; **334**(7594): 635–6.

Tabor A, Watt HC, Wald NJ. Endometrial thickness as a test for endometrial cancer in women with postmenopausal vaginal bleeding. *Obstet Gynecol*. 2002; **99**(4): 663–70.

Tahir MM, Bigrigg MA, Browning JJ, *et al*. A randomised controlled trial comparing transvaginal ultrasound, outpatient hysteroscopy and endometrial biopsy with inpatient hysteroscopy and curettage. *Br J Obstet Gynaecol*. 1999; **106**(12): 1259–64.

van Dongen H, de Kroon CD, Jacobi CE, *et al*. Diagnostic hysteroscopy in abnormal uterine bleeding: a systematic review and meta-analysis. *BJOG*. 2007; **114**(6): 664–75.

20

PROSTATIC HYPERTROPHY

Benign prostatic hyperplasia 1

Which therapy?

Assess: • urinary symptoms, preferably using a validated questionnaire such as the International Prostate Symptom Score (IPSS). • sexual symptoms (e.g. erectile dysfunction, pain/discomfort on ejaculation).	• Address any concerns the man may have about the possibility of prostate cancer. • Discuss the advantages and disadvantages of prostate-specific antigen (PSA) testing.	• Discuss methods for coping with urinary symptoms.

Treatment choice

Predominantly determined by patient preference, following discussion of expected benefits and risks of treatment

If lower urinary tract symptoms (LUTS) are not bothersome (i.e. minimal frequency, nocturia, urgency, and urge incontinence) and there are no risk factors for progression (large prostate, or men raised PSA).	Watchful waiting is appropriate
Men with bothersome moderate-to-severe symptoms	Medical treatment is generally recommended
Men with 'mild' symptoms that are of significant 'bother'	May request a treatment trial of medical treatment
If LUTS are not bothersome, but risk factors for progression are present, e.g. enlarged prostate on digital rectal examination	Consider a 5-alpha reductase inhibitor (finasteride or dutasteride). Symptomatic improvement occurs in most men 3 to 6 months after initiation
If LUTS are bothersome and risk factors for progression are present	Consider an alpha-blocker, or a 5-alpha reductase inhibitor, or both drugs combined. With combination therapy, consider stopping the alpha-blocker at 6 months except in men with severe symptoms for whom surgery would be undesirable
If LUTS are bothersome, prostate obstruction is present and there are no risk factors for progression	An alpha blocker (alfuzosin, doxazosin, prazosin, tamsulosin, or terazosin) is drug of first choice. Symptoms should improve within several days, with full response after 4 to 6 weeks. Choice of a particular alpha blocker depends on safety, convenience, and cost
Surgery is generally reserved for men who have failed to respond to medical treatments or who have developed complications	*For recommendations regarding referral of men with lower urinary tract symptoms, see NICE referral guide at www.nice.org.uk/nicemedia/pdf/Referraladvice.pdf*

Practical prescribing points

For further information please see the Medicines Compendium (www.medicines.org.uk) or the British National Formulary (www.bnf.org).

Alpha blockers

• Avoid alpha blockers in men with a history of postural hypotension or micturition syncope.
• Alpha blockers are best taken at bedtime, especially starting dose, as there is a risk of first-dose and postural hypotension (except for tamsulosin), particularly in elderly people and those already taking antihypertensive drug treatment.
• Adverse effects are usually minor and mainly of a vasodilatory or central nervous system type. They tend to be dose-related and are often either tolerated or disappear with continued use.
• Modified-release alfuzosin, doxazosin, and tamsulosin have been reported as having less vasodilatory-type adverse effects, e.g. dizziness and first-dose antihypertension, than standard-release preparations. Modified-release formulations therefore do not require dose titration.

5-alpha reductase inhibitors

• Sexual adverse effects, including decreased libido, ejaculation disorder and erectile dysfunction, may be experienced by some men.
• However, in general finasteride and dutasteride are well tolerated – people experience less adverse effects than with alpha blockers.
• Men taking finasteride or dutasteride who have partners of child-bearing age are advised to use a condom to avoid a very slight chance of foetal abnormalities to male genitalia. Also women of child-bearing age should not handle the drug preparations.

Benign prostatic hyperplasia 2

Investigate?

Lower urinary tract symptoms

Consider tests to exclude complications or other causes of lower urinary tract symptoms
- Serum creatinine: to exclude renal impairment and to establish a baseline level.
- Urinalysis: to check for blood, leucocytes, nitrite, glucose.
  - Nitrite and leucocytes may indicate urinary tract infection (UTI).
  - Blood may indicate bladder carcinoma as a cause of lower urinary tract symptoms.
  - Glucose may indicate diabetes mellitus.
- Urine culture: to exclude UTI.

Prostate-specific antigen testing

- There is no consensus on whether men with lower urinary tract symptoms should opt in or opt out of prostate-specific antigen (PSA) testing – a decision should be made on an individual basis following counselling regarding the pros and cons of testing.
- Before having a PSA test the man should not have:
  - an active urinary tract infection
  - ejaculated in the previous 48 hours
  - exercised vigorously in the last 48 hours
  - had a prostate biopsy in the previous 6 weeks.
- The PSA test should be done before the digital rectal examination. If this is not practicable, it is recommended that the PSA test be delayed a week.

Follow-up advice

- If watchful waiting is undertaken, review at least every 12 months.
- The International Prostate Symptom Score (I-PSS) assesses severity of symptoms and their impact on an individual. It is a valuable tool for monitoring progress and response to treatment.
- Follow up alpha blocker response about 6 to 12 weeks after starting treatment. If a man has little or no apparent benefit with an alpha blocker, try increasing the dose of alpha-blocker, or try adding a 5-alpha reductase inhibitor if the prostate is large.
- In men on combination therapy, expert opinion is that the alpha blocker should be stopped after 6 months, except in men with severe symptoms and for whom surgery would be undesirable.

International Prostate Symptom Score (I-PSS)

	Not at all	Less than one time in five	Less than half the time	About half the time	More than half the time	Almost always
Over the past month, how often have you had a sensation of not emptying your bladder completely after you finished urinating?	0	1	2	3	4	5
Over the past month, how often have you had to urinate again less than two hours after you first urinated?	0	1	2	3	4	5
Over the past month, how often have you found you stopped and started again several times when you urinated?	0	1	2	3	4	5
Over the past month, how often have you found it difficult to postpone urination?	0	1	2	3	4	5
Over the past month, how many times have you had to push or strain to begin urination?	0	1	2	3	4	5
Over the past month, how often have you had a weak urinary stream?	0	1	2	3	4	5

	None	Once	Twice	x Three	x Four	≥Five
Over the past month, how many times did you most typically urinate, from the time you went to bed at night to the time you got up in the morning?	0	1	2	3	4	5

Quality of life due to urinary symptoms

If you were to spend the rest of your life with your urinary condition just the way it is now, how would you feel about that?	Delighted	0
	Pleased	1
	Mostly satisfied	2
	Mixed (about equally satisfied/dissatisfied)	3
	Mostly dissatisfied	4
	Unhappy	5
	Terrible	6

This single question is recommended to assess the patient's own view of his quality of life. The question can be used to initiate a discussion).

I-PSS severity of symptoms score

The I-PSS has been developed to help evaluate the severity of symptoms caused by BPH. For each of the seven questions, patients should assign a score from 0 to 5. These scores should be added together, giving a total I-PSS score of between 0 and 35.

Severity of symptoms
Mild = 0 to 7
Moderate = 8 to 19
Severe = 20 to 35
It is recommended that the I-PSS score and quality of life question be used and recorded at the initial consultation and after treatment to monitor progress.

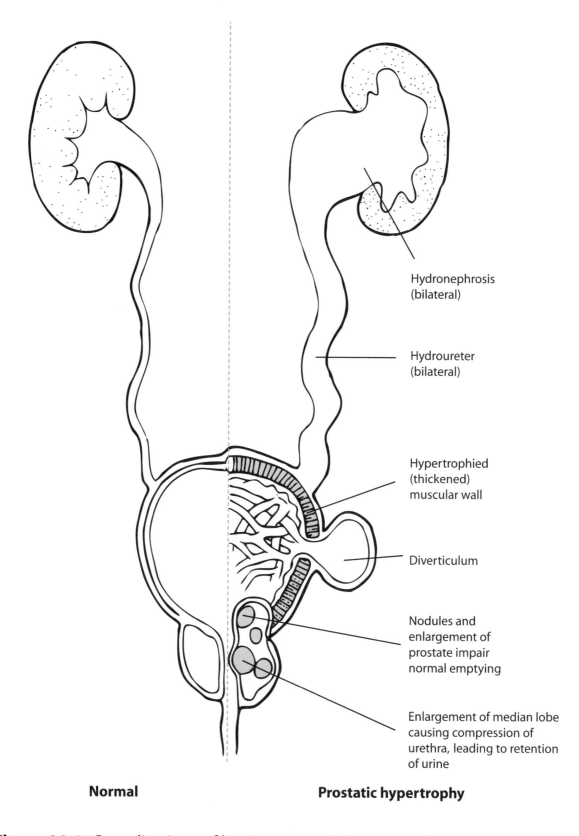

Hydronephrosis
(bilateral)

Hydroureter
(bilateral)

Hypertrophied
(thickened)
muscular wall

Diverticulum

Nodules and
enlargement of
prostate impair
normal emptying

Enlargement of median lobe
causing compression of
urethra, leading to retention
of urine

Normal **Prostatic hypertrophy**

Figure 20.1 Complications of benign prostatic hypertrophy

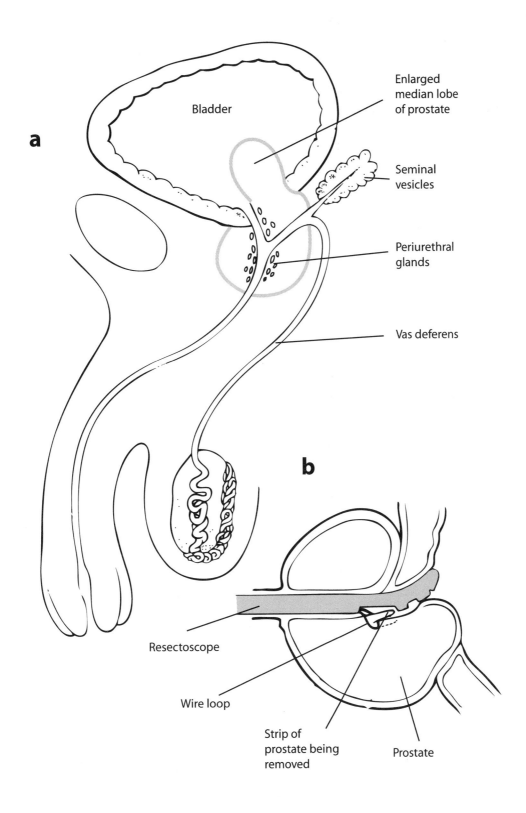

Figure 20.2 a: Enlarged prostate; b: Removal of hypertrophied prostate with resectoscope

Benign prostatic hypertrophy references

These guidelines are an extract from the excellent online primary care resource: Clinical Knowledge Summaries service www.cks.library.nhs.uk (the successor to PRODIGY). Clinical Summary: Benign Prostatic Hypertrophy. Available at: www.cks.library.nhs. uk/prostate_benign_hyperplasia#-221806
Reproduced with permission.

de la Rosette J, Madersbacher S, Alivizatos G, *et al*. EAU Guidelines on Benign Prostatic Hyperplasia. Arnhem: European Association of Urology; 2004. Available at: www.uroweb.org/fileadmin/tx_eauguidelines/BPH.pdf

Department of Health. *Prostate Cancer Risk Management Programme: Reference Booklet.* London: DH; 2002. Available at: www.cancerscreening.nhs.uk/prostate/prostate-booklet-text.pdf

Edwards JE, Moore RA. Finasteride in the treatment of clinical benign prostatic hyperplasia: a systematic review of randomised trials. *BMC Urol.* 2002; **2**(1): 14.

Jacobsen SJ, Jacobson DJ, Girman CJ, *et al*. Natural history of prostatism: risk factors for acute urinary retention. *J Urol* 1997; **158**(2): 481–7.

Madersbacher S, Alivizatos G, Nordling J, *et al*. EAU guidelines on assessment, therapy and follow-up of men with lower urinary tract symptoms suggestive of benign prostatic obstruction. *Eur Urol.* 2004; **46**(5): 547–54.

McVary KT. Alfuzosin for symptomatic benign prostatic hyperplasia: long-term experience. *J Urol.* 2006; **175**(1): 35–42.

Patel AK, Chapple CR. Benign prostatic hyperplasia: treatment in primary care. *BMJ.* 2006; **333**(7567): 535–9.

Speakman MJ, Kirby RS, Joyce A, *et al*. Guideline for the primary care management of male lower urinary tract symptoms. *BJU Int.* 2004; **93**(7): 985–90.

Wilt TJ, MacDonald R, Rutks I. Tamsulosin for benign prostatic hyperplasia. *Cochrane Database Rev.* 2002; **4**: CD002081.

Wilt TJ, N'Dow J. Benign prostatic hyperplasia. Part 2 – management. *BMJ.* 2008; **336**(7637): 206–10.

21

SORE THROAT

Sore throat

Diagnosis of acute sore throat

Clinical examination should not be relied upon to differentiate between viral and bacterial sore throat **B**	Throat swabs or rapid antigen testing should not be carried out routinely in sore throat **B**

Management of acute sore throat

Sore throat associated with stridor or respiratory difficulty is an absolute indication for admission to hospital **C**

Paracetamol is the drug of choice for analgesia in sore throat **C**	Routine use of non-steroidal anti-inflammatory drugs (NSAIDs) is not recommended **B**

Antibiotics & acute sore throat

There is insufficient evidence to support the routine use of antibiotics in acute sore throat

Antibiotics should *not* be used:

For symptomatic relief **A**	Specifically to prevent the development of rheumatic fever or glomerulonephritis **B**
Routinely to prevent cross infection in the general population **B**	Specifically to prevent suppurative complications **C**

In severe cases, where the practitioner is concerned about the clinical condition of the patient, antibiotics should not be withheld ☑

Indications for tonsillectomy

Patients should meet all of the following criteria: Sore throats are due to tonsillitis Five or more episodes of sore throat per year Symptoms for at least a year Episodes of sore throat are disabling and prevent normal functioning **C**	Following specialist referral, a six-month period of watchful waiting is recommended to establish the pattern of symptoms and allow the patient to consider the implications of the operation **C**
	Once a decision is made for tonsillectomy, this should be performed as soon as possible to maximise the period of benefit **B**

Key: **A B C D** Indicates grade of evidence	☑ Good practice point

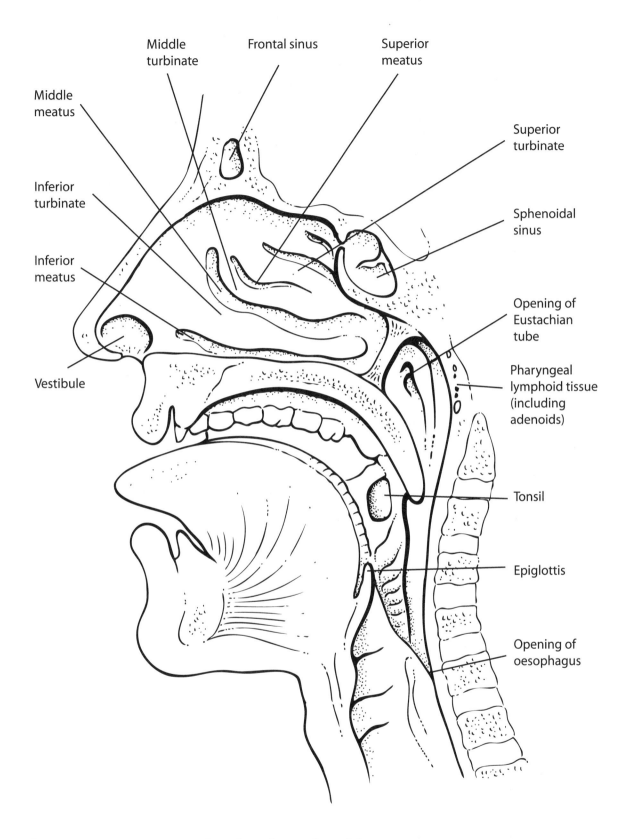

Figure 21.1 Anatomy of oral and nasal cavities

Middle turbinate

Frontal sinus

Superior meatus

Middle meatus

Inferior turbinate

Inferior meatus

Vestibule

Superior turbinate

Sphenoidal sinus

Opening of Eustachian tube

Pharyngeal lymphoid tissue (including adenoids)

Tonsil

Epiglottis

Opening of oesophagus

Sore throat references

This guideline is an extract from the quick reference guide to:
Scottish Intercollegiate Guidelines Network. *Management of Sore Throat and Indications for Tonsillectomy: a national clinical guideline 34*. Edinburgh: SIGN; 1999. Available at: www.sign.ac.uk/pdf/qrg34.pdf

Burton MJ, Towler B, Glasziou P. Tonsillectomy versus non-surgical treatment for chronic/recurrent acute tonsillitis. *Cochrane Database Syst Rev.* 1999; **3**: CD001802.

Butler CC, Rollnick S, Pill R, *et al*. Understanding the culture of prescribing: qualitative study of general practitioners' and patients' perceptions of antibiotics for sore throats. *BMJ*. 1998; **317**(7159): 637–42.

Cooper RJ, Hoffman JR, Bartlett JG, *et al*. Principles of appropriate antibiotic use for acute pharyngitis in adults: background. *Ann Intern Med*. 2001; **134**(6): 509–17.

Del Mar C, Glasziou P. Upper respiratory tract infection. *Clin Evid*. 2003; **6** (9): 1701–11

Del Mar CB, Glasziou PP, Spinks AB. Antibiotics for sore throat. *Cochrane Database Syst Rev.* 2006: **18**(4): CD000023.

Department of Health. *The Path of Least Resistance*. London: DH and the Standing Medical Advisory Committee (SMAC); 1998. Available at: www.advisorybodies.doh.gov.uk/pub/docs/doh/smacrep.pdf

Little P, Gould C, Williamson I, *et al*. Reattendance and complications in a randomised trial of prescribing strategies for sore throat: the medicalising effect of prescribing antibiotics. *BMJ*. 1997; **315**(7104): 350–2.

Little P, Williamson I. Sore throat management in general practice. *Fam Pract*. 1996; **13**(3): 317–21.

McKerrow, W. *Tonsillitis*. London: BMJ Clinical Evidence; 2006.

Schaad UB. Acute streptococcal tonsillopharyngitis: a review of clinical efficacy and bacteriological eradication. *J Int Med Res*. 2004; **32**(1): 1–13.

22

STROKE

Primary care concise stroke guidelines 1

Stroke is a major cause of mortality and morbidity in the United Kingdom, affecting over 130,000 people each year. Much of the responsibility for delivering effective secondary prevention and managing longer-term problems associated with stroke falls to the primary care team. These guidelines are selected from the full National Clinical Guidelines for Stroke as being the key ones that primary care teams need to be aware of, although they are not the only guidelines relevant to primary care. They apply to all patients with TIA and stroke, irrespective of whether it is a first or recurrent stroke.

Investigation and management of patients with TIA

The risk of developing a stroke after a hemispheric TIA can be as high as 20% within the first month, with the greatest risk within the first 72 hours.

- Patients with TIA, or patients with a stroke who have made a good recovery when seen, should be assessed and investigated in a specialist service (e.g. neurovascular clinic) as soon as possible within 7 days of the incident.
- Once all symptoms have resolved after TIA, aspirin (at an initial dose of 300 mg daily) should be prescribed immediately and continued until a definitive management plan is established.
- Patients with more than one TIA in a week should be investigated in hospital immediately.

Acute stroke management

- Patients should be admitted to hospital for initial care and treatment, with the expectation that they will be managed on a stroke unit. Exceptions may include those relatively few patients for whom the diagnosis will make no difference to management, e.g. where optimal management is palliative care.
- Patients should only be managed at home if the guidelines for acute investigation, treatment and care can be adhered to.
- Patients with persisting impairments not admitted to hospital should be seen by a specialist stroke rehabilitation team that includes a specialist occupational therapist.
- Brain imaging should be undertaken as soon as possible in all patients, at least within 24 hours of onset, unless there are good clinical reasons for not doing so.
- Brain imaging should be undertaken as a matter of urgency if the patient:
    - is currently taking anticoagulant treatment
    - has a depressed level of consciousness
    - has papilloedema, neck stiffness or fever
    - has indications for thrombolysis or early anticoagulation.
    - has a known bleeding tendency
    - has unexplained progressive or fluctuating symptoms
    - has severe headache at onset
- All stroke patients should have access to specialist palliative care expertise when needed.

Secondary prevention of stroke and TIA

Patients who have suffered a stroke remain at an increased risk of a further stroke (between 30 and 43% risk within five years). Patients with TIA and stroke also have an increased risk of myocardial infarction and other vascular events. The risk of further stroke is highest early after stroke or TIA. Therefore, there should be a high priority given to rapid delivery of evidence-based secondary prevention.

General
- All patients should have an individualised strategy for stroke prevention that should be implemented within a maximum of 7 days of acute stroke or TIA.
- All patients should be given appropriate advice on lifestyle factors, including: stopping smoking, regular exercise, diet, achieving a satisfactory weight, reducing the intake of salt and avoiding excess alcohol.
- All patients should receive regular review and treatment of risk factors for vascular disease for the rest of their lives after a stroke, with inclusion on a stroke register and a minimum of annual follow-up.
- All patients should receive an annual flu vaccination.

Primary care concise stroke guidelines 2

Secondary prevention of stroke and TIA (cont.)

Blood pressure
- All patients should have their blood pressure checked, and high blood pressure persisting for over 2 weeks should be treated. The British Hypertension Society guidelines are: in non-diabetic people with hypertension, the optimal blood pressure treatment goals are systolic blood pressure <140 mmHg and diastolic blood pressure <85 mmHg; for patients with diabetes mellitus and high blood pressure, the optimal goals of control are 130/80.
- Further reduction of blood pressure should be undertaken using a thiazide diuretic (e.g. bendroflumethiazide or indapamide) or an ACE inhibitor (e.g. perindopril or ramipril) or preferably a combination of both, unless there are contraindications.

Anti-thrombotic treatment
- All patients with ischaemic stroke or TIA who are not on anticoagulation should be taking an antiplatelet agent, i.e. low-dose aspirin (e.g. 75mg), or clopidogrel, or a combination of low-dose aspirin and dipyridamole modified release (MR). Where patients are aspirin intolerant an alternative antiplatelet agent (e.g. clopidogrel 75mg daily or dipyridamole MR 200mg twice daily) should be used.
- Anticoagulation should be started in every patient with persistent or paroxysmal atrial fibrillation (valvular or non-valvular), unless contraindicated.
- Anticoagulants should not be used for patients in sinus rhythm unless there is a major source of cardiac embolism.
- Anticoagulants should not be started until brain imaging has excluded haemorrhage, and usually not until 14 days have passed from the onset of an ischaemic stroke.

Anti-lipid agents
- Treatment with a statin (e.g. 40mg simvastatin) should be given to patients with ischaemic stroke or TIA, and total cholesterol of >3.5mmol/l unless contraindicated.

Longer-term management

By 6 months, over half of stroke survivors will need some help with activities of daily living. 15% will have communication impairments and 53% will have motor weakness, and many will have problems with mood or cognition.
Morbidity within the carers is high.

- Patients and their carers should have their individual psychosocial and support needs reviewed on a regular basis. This will include mood (depression and anxiety), cognitive impairment, pain, communication difficulties, continence, functional ability, equipment needs and social integration.
- Patients should continue to have access to specialist care and rehabilitation after leaving hospital.
- Any patient with reduced function at 6 months or later after stroke should be assessed for a period of further targeted rehabilitation.
- Independence should be encouraged. As patients become more active, consideration should be given to withdrawal of physical and psychological support, enteral tubes, cessation of therapy and withdrawal of personal support.

Information and support needs
- The needs of the carers should be considered from the outset.
- Health and social services professionals should ensure that patients and their families have information about the statutory and voluntary organisations offering services specific to these needs.

Audit
- All GPs should keep a register of stroke patients and conduct a regular audit of secondary prevention and management of chronic disability, as specified in the new GMS contract.

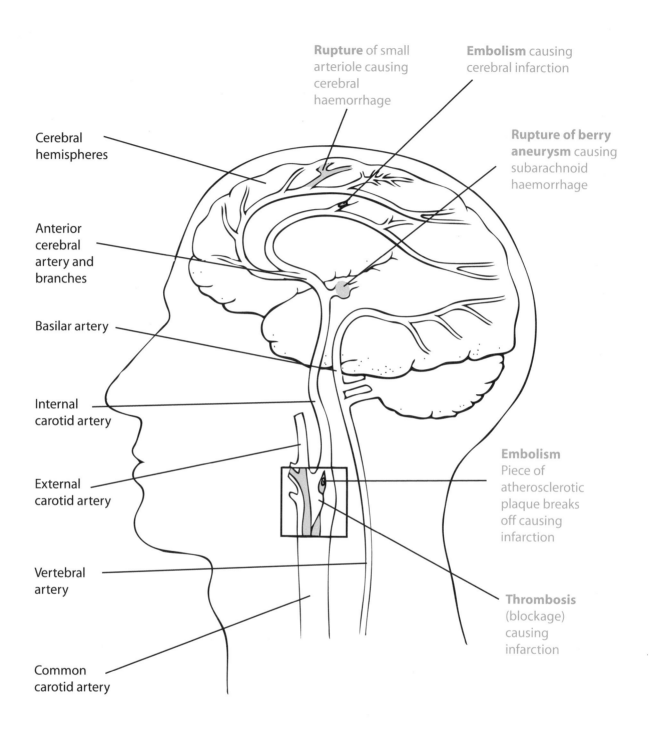

Rupture of small arteriole causing cerebral haemorrhage

Embolism causing cerebral infarction

Rupture of berry aneurysm causing subarachnoid haemorrhage

Cerebral hemispheres

Anterior cerebral artery and branches

Basilar artery

Internal carotid artery

External carotid artery

Embolism Piece of atherosclerotic plaque breaks off causing infarction

Vertebral artery

Thrombosis (blockage) causing infarction

Common carotid artery

Figure 22.1 How hypertension can cause strokes

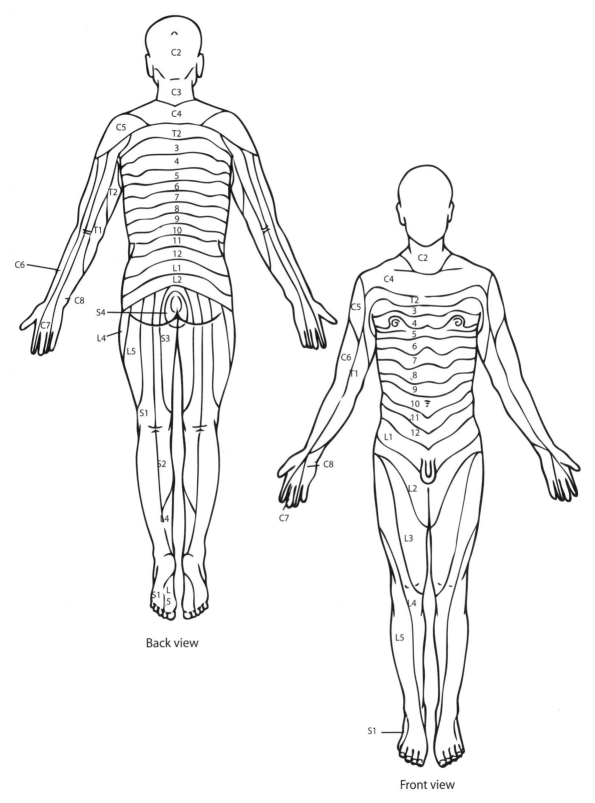

Figure 22.2 Dermatomes

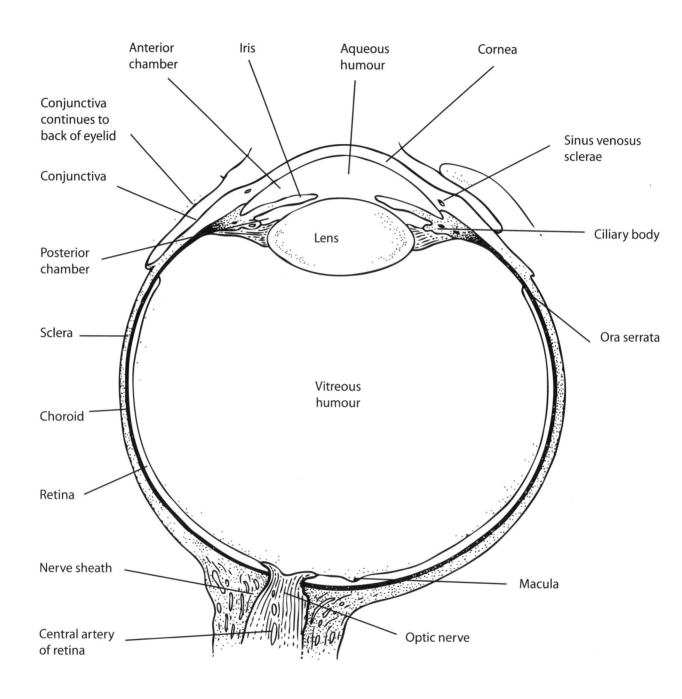

Figure 22.3 Structure of the eye

Stroke references

This guideline is reproduced from:

The Intercollegiate Working Party for Stroke, Royal College of Physicians. *Primary Care Concise Guidelines for Stroke.* 2nd edn. London: RCP; 2004. Available at: www.rcplondon.ac.uk/pubs/books/stroke/stroke_primarycare_2ed.pdf

Amarenco P, Lavallee P, Touboul PJ. Stroke prevention, blood cholesterol, and statins. *Lancet Neurol.* 2004; **3**(5): 271–8.

CAPRIE Steering Committee. A randomised, blinded, trial of clopidogrel versus aspirin in patients at risk of ischaemic events (CAPRIE). *Lancet.* 1996; **348**(9038): 1329–39.

Cohen SN. Preventing recurrent ischemic stroke: a 3-step plan. *J Fam Pract.* 2005; **54**(5): 412–22.

Department of Health. *National Service Framework for Coronary Heart Disease.* London: DH; 2000. Available at: www.dh.gov.uk/en/Publicationsandstatistics/Publications/PublicationsPolicyAndGuidance/DH_4094275

The European/Australasian Stroke Prevention in Reversible Ischaemia Trial (ESPRIT) Study Group. Aspirin plus dipyridamole versus aspirin alone after cerebral ischaemia of arterial origin (ESPRIT): randomised controlled trial. *Lancet.* 2006; **367**(9523): 1665–73.

Hankey GJ, Eikelboom JW. Adding aspirin to clopidogrel after TIA and ischemic stroke: benefits do not match risks [review]. *Neurol.* 2005; **64**(7): 1117–21.

Lee CD, Folsom AR, Blair SN. Physical activity and stroke risk: a meta-analysis. *Stroke.* 2003; **34**(10): 2475–81.

Nguyen-Huynh MN, Johnston SC. Transient ischemic attack: a neurologic emergency. *Curr Neurol Neurosci Rep.* 2005; **5**(1): 13–20.

Rothwell PM, Giles MF, Flossmann E, *et al.* A simple score (ABCD) to identify individuals at high early risk of stroke after transient ischaemic attack. *Lancet.* 2005; **366**(9479): 29–36.

Rothwell PMM, Warlow CPM. Timing of TIAs preceding stroke: time window for prevention is very short. *Neurol* 2005; **64**(5): 817–20.

23

SUSPECTED CANCER

Lung

Immediate referral
Consider immediate referral for patients with:
• signs of superior vena caval obstruction (swelling of the face/neck with fixed elevation of jugular venous pressure)
• stridor.

Urgent referral
Urgently refer patients with:
• persistent haemoptysis (in smokers or ex-smokers aged 40 years and older)
• a chest X-ray suggestive of lung cancer (including pleural effusion and slowly resolving consolidation)
• a normal chest X-ray where there is a high suspicion of lung cancer
• a history of asbestos exposure and recent onset of chest pain, shortness of breath or unexplained systemic symptoms where a chest X-ray indicates pleural effusion, pleural mass or any suspicious lung pathology.

Urgent chest X-ray
Urgently refer for chest X-ray (the report should be returned within 5 days) for patients with any of the following:
• haemoptysis
• unexplained or persistent (longer than 3 weeks):
  – chest and/or shoulder pain
  – dyspnoea
  – weight loss
  – chest signs
  – hoarseness
  – finger clubbing
  – cervical or supraclavicular lymph adenopathy
  – cough
  – features suggestive of metastasis from a lung cancer (for example, secondaries in the brain, bone, liver, skin).
• underlying chronic respiratory problems with unexplained changes in existing symptoms.

Upper GI

Urgent referral for endoscopy/referral to specialist
Urgently refer for endoscopy, or to a specialist, patients of any age with dyspepsia and any of the following:
• chronic gastrointestinal bleeding
• dysphagia
• progressive unintentional weight loss
• persistent vomiting
• iron deficiency anaemia
• epigastric mass
• suspicious barium meal result.

Urgent referral
Urgently refer patients presenting with:
• dysphagia
• unexplained upper abdominal pain and weight loss, with or without back pain
• upper abdominal mass without dyspepsia
• obstructive jaundice (depending on clinical state) – consider urgent ultrasound if available.

Consider urgent referral for patients presenting with:
• persistent vomiting and weight loss in the absence of dyspepsia
• unexplained weight loss or iron deficiency anaemia in the absence of dyspepsia
• unexplained worsening of dyspepsia and:
  – Barrett's oesophagus
  – known dysplasia, atrophic gastritis or intestinal metaplasia
  – peptic ulcer surgery over 20 years ago.

Urgent endoscopy
Urgently refer for endoscopy patients aged 55 years and older with unexplained and persistent recent-onset dyspepsia alone.

Note that for patients under 55 years, referral for endoscopy is not necessary in the absence of alarm symptoms.

Lower GI

Urgent referral
Urgently refer patients:
• aged 40 years and older, reporting rectal bleeding with a change of bowel habit towards looser stools and/or increased stool frequency persisting 6 weeks or more
• aged 60 years and older, with rectal bleeding persisting for 6 weeks or more without a change in bowel habit and without anal symptoms
• aged 60 years and older, with a change in bowel habit to looser stools and/or more frequent stools persisting for 6 weeks or more without rectal bleeding
• of any age with a right lower abdominal mass consistent with involvement of the large bowel
• of any age with a palpable rectal mass (intraluminal and not pelvic; a pelvic mass outside the bowel would warrant an urgent referral to a urologist or gynaecologist)
• who are men of any age with unexplained iron deficiency anaemia and a haemoglobin of 11g/100ml or below
• who are non-menstruating women with unexplained iron deficiency anaemia and a haemoglobin of 10g/100ml or below.

In a patient with equivocal symptoms who is not unduly anxious, it is reasonable to 'treat, watch and wait'.

Breast

Urgent referral
Urgently refer patients:
• of any age with a discrete, hard lump with fixation, with or without skin tethering
• who are female, aged 30 years and older with a discrete lump that persists after their next period, or presents after menopause
• who are female, aged younger than 30 years:
  – with a lump that enlarges
  – with a lump that is fixed and hard
  – in whom there are other reasons for concern such as family history.
• of any age, with previous breast cancer, who present with a further lump or suspicious symptoms
• with unilateral eczematous skin or nipple change that does not respond to topical treatment
• with nipple distortion of recent onset
• with spontaneous unilateral bloody nipple discharge
• who are male, aged 50 years and older with a unilateral, firm subareolar mass with or without nipple distortion or associated skin changes.

Non-urgent referral
Consider non-urgent referral in:
• women aged younger than 30 years with a lump
• patients with breast pain and no palpable abnormality, when initial treatment fails and/or with unexplained persistent symptoms. (Use of mammography in these patients is not recommended.)

Gynaecological

Urgent referral
Urgently refer patients:
- with clinical features suggestive of cervical cancer on examination. A smear test is not required before referral, and a previous negative result should not delay referral
- not on hormone replacement therapy with post-menopausal bleeding
- on hormone replacement therapy with persistent or unexplained post-menopausal bleeding after cessation of hormone replacement therapy for 6 weeks
- taking tamoxifen with post-menopausal bleeding
- with an unexplained vulval lump
- with vulval bleeding due to ulceration.

Consider urgent referral for patients with persistent intermenstrual bleeding and negative pelvic examination.

Urgently refer for an ultrasound scan patients with a palpable abdominal or pelvic mass on examination that is not obviously uterine fibroids or not of gastrointestinal or urological origin. If the scan is suggestive of cancer, an urgent referral should be made. If urgent ultrasound is not available, an urgent referral should be made.

Urological

Prostate
Urgently refer patients:
- with a hard, irregular prostate typical of a prostate carcinoma. Prostate specific antigen (PSA) should be measured and the result should accompany the referral. (An urgent referral is not needed if the prostate is simply enlarged and the PSA is in the age-specific reference range.)
- with a normal prostate, but rising/raised age-specific PSA, with or without lower urinary tract symptoms (in patients compromised by other comorbidities, a discussion with the patient or carers and/or a specialist may be more appropriate).
- with symptoms and high PSA levels.

The age-specific cut-off PSA measurements recommended by the Prostate Cancer Risk Management Programme are as follows:
- aged 50–59 ≥3.0ng/ml;
- aged 60–69 ≥4.0ng/ml;
- aged 70 and over ≥5.0ng/ml.
(Note that there are no age-specific reference ranges for men over 80 years. Nearly all men of this age have at least a focus of cancer in the prostate. Prostate cancer only needs to be diagnosed in this age group if it is likely to need palliative treatment.)

Bladder and renal
Urgently refer patients:
- of any age with painless macroscopic haematuria
- aged 40 years and older who present with recurrent or persistent urinary tract infection associated with haematuria
- aged 50 years and older who are found to have unexplained microscopic haematuria
- with an abdominal mass identified clinically or on imaging that is thought to arise from the urinary tract.

Testicular
Urgently refer patients with a swelling or mass in the body of the testis. Consider an urgent ultrasound in men with a scrotal mass that does not transilluminate and/or when the body of the testis cannot be distinguished.

Penile
Urgently refer patients with symptoms or signs of penile cancer. These include progressive ulceration or a mass in the glans or prepuce particularly, but can involve the skin of the penile shaft. (Lumps within the corpora cavernosa can indicate Peyronie's disease, which does not require urgent referral.)

Non-urgent referral
Non-urgently refer patients under 50 years of age with microscopic haematuria. Patients with proteinuria or raised serum creatinine should be referred to a renal physician. If there is no proteinuria and serum creatinine is normal, a non-urgent referral to a urologist should be made.

Haematological

Immediate referral
Immediately refer patients:
- with a blood count/film reported as acute leukaemia
- with spinal cord compression or renal failure suspected of being caused by myeloma.

Urgent referral
Urgently refer patients with unexplained splenomegaly

Combinations of the following symptoms and signs warrant full examination, further investigation (including a blood count and film) and possible referral:
- fatigue
- drenching night sweats
- fever
- weight loss
- generalised itching
- breathlessness
- bruising
- bleeding
- recurrent infections
- bone pain
- alcohol-induced pain
- abdominal pain
- lymphadenopathy
- splenomegaly.

The urgency of referral depends on the symptom severity and findings of investigations.

Skin

Melanoma
Diagnosis
Change is a key element in diagnosing malignant melanoma. For low-suspicion lesions, undertake careful monitoring for change using the 7-point checklist for assessment of pigmented skin lesions (see below) for 8 weeks. Make measurements with photographs and a marker scale and/or ruler.

Major features of lesions:
- change in size
- irregular shape
- irregular colour.

Minor features of lesions:
- largest diameter ≥7mm
- inflammation
- oozing
- change in sensation.

Lesions scoring 3 points or more (based on major features scoring 2 points each and minor features scoring 1 point each) in the 7-point checklist above are suspicious. (If you strongly suspect cancer, any one feature is adequate to prompt urgent referral.)

Urgent referal
Urgently refer patients:
- with a lesion suspected to be melanoma. (Excision in primary care should be avoided.)

Squamous cell carcinomas
Urgently refer patients:
- with non-healing keratinising or crusted tumours larger than 1cm with significant induration on palpation. They are commonly found on the face, scalp or back of the hand.
- with a documented expansion over 8 weeks
- who have had an organ transplant and develop new or growing cutaneous lesions, as squamous cell carcinoma is common with immunosuppression but may be atypical and aggressive
- with histological diagnosis of a squamous cell carcinoma.

Non-urgent referral
Basal cell carcinomas
Basal cell carcinomas are slow growing, usually without significant expansion over 2 months, and usually occur on the face. If basal cell carcinoma is suspected, refer non-urgently.

Head and neck and thyroid

Head and neck
Urgent referral
Urgently refer patients with:
- an unexplained lump in the neck of recent onset, or a previously undiagnosed lump that has changed over a period of 3 to 6 weeks
- an unexplained persistent swelling in the parotid or submandibular gland
- an unexplained persistent sore or painful throat
- unilateral unexplained pain in the head and neck area for more than 4 weeks, associated with otalgia (ear ache) but a normal otoscopy
- unexplained ulceration of the oral mucosa or mass persisting for more than 3 weeks
- unexplained red and white patches of the oral mucosa that are painful or swollen or bleeding (including suspected lichen planus).

For patients with persistent symptoms or signs related to the oral cavity in whom a definitive diagnosis of a benign lesion cannot be made, refer or follow up until the symptoms and signs disappear. If the symptoms and signs have not disappeared after 6 weeks, make an urgent referral.

To a dentist
Urgently refer to a dentist patients with unexplained tooth mobility persisting for more than 3 weeks.
Monitor for oral cancer patients with confirmed oral lichen planus, as part of routine dental examination.
Advise all patients, including those with dentures, to have regular dental checkups.

For a chest X-ray
Urgently refer for chest X-ray patients with hoarseness persisting for more than 3 weeks, particularly smokers aged older than 50 years and heavy drinkers.

If there is a positive finding, urgently refer to a team specialising in the management of lung cancer. If there is a negative finding, urgently refer to a team specialising in head and neck cancer.

Non-urgent referral
Non-urgently refer a patient with unexplained red and white patches of the oral mucosa that are not painful, swollen or bleeding (including suspected lichen planus).

Thyroid cancer
Immediate referral
Immediately refer patients with symptoms of tracheal compression including stridor due to thyroid swelling.

Urgent referral
Urgently refer patients with a thyroid swelling associated with any of the following:
- a solitary nodule increasing in size
- a history of neck irradiation
- a family history of an endocrine tumour
- unexplained hoarseness or voice changes
- cervical lymphadenopathy
- very young (pre-pubertal) patient
- patient aged 65 years and older.

Bone and sarcoma

Bone tumours
Immediate X-ray
Refer for an immediate X-ray a patient with a suspected spontaneous fracture.
If the X-ray:
- indicates possible bone cancer, urgently refer
- is normal but symptoms persist, follow up and/or request repeat X-ray, bone function tests or referral.

Soft tissue sarcomas
Urgent referral
Urgently refer if a patient presents with a palpable lump that is:
- greater than about 5 cm in diameter
- deep to fascia, fixed or immobile
- increasing in size
- painful
- a recurrence after previous excision.
If a patient has HIV, consider Kaposi's sarcoma and make an urgent referral if suspected.

Urgent investigation
Urgently investigate increasing, unexplained or persistent bone pain or tenderness, particularly pain at rest (and especially if not in the joint), or an unexplained limp. In older people metastases, myeloma or lymphoma, as well as sarcoma, should be considered.

Brain and CNS

Urgent referral
Urgently refer patients with:
- symptoms related to the CNS, including:
  - progressive neurological deficit
  - new-onset seizures or headaches
  - mental changes
  - cranial nerve palsy
  - unilateral sensorineural deafness in whom a brain tumour is suspected
- headaches of recent onset accompanied by features suggestive of raised intracranial pressure, for example:
  - vomiting or drowsiness
  - posture-related headache
  - pulse-synchronous tinnitus or other focal or non-focal neurological symptoms, for example black-out, change in personality or memory
- a new, qualitatively different, unexplained headache that becomes progressively severe
- suspected recent-onset seizures (refer to neurologist).

Consider urgent referral (to an appropriate specialist) in patients with rapid progression of:
- subacute focal neurological deficit
- unexplained cognitive impairment, behavioural disturbance or slowness, or a combination of these
- personality changes confirmed by a witness and for which there is no reasonable explanation even in the absence of the other symptoms and signs of a brain tumour.

Risk factors
Urgently refer patients previously diagnosed with any cancer who develop any of the following symptoms:
- recent onset seizures
- progressive neurological deficit
- persistent headaches
- new mental or cognitive changes
- new neurological changes

Non-urgent referral
Consider non-urgent referral or discussion with specialist for:
- unexplained headaches of recent onset that are:
  - present for at least 1 month
  - not accompanied by features suggestive of raised intracranial pressure.

Cancer in children and young people

General
Consider referral
Consider referral when a child or young person presents with persistent back pain (an examination is needed and a full blood count and blood film). Persistent parental anxiety is sufficient reason for referral, even where a benign cause is considered most likely. Take into account parental insight and knowledge when considering urgent referral.

Urgent referral
Urgently refer when a child or young person presents several times (for example, three or more times) with the same problem, but with no clear diagnosis (investigations should also be carried out).

There are associations between Down's syndrome and leukaemia, between neurofibromatosis and CNS tumours, and between other rare syndromes and some cancers. Be alert to the potential significance of unexplained symptoms in children with such syndromes.

Brain and CNS tumours
Immediate referral
Immediately refer children or young people with:
- a reduced level of consciousness
- headache and vomiting that cause early morning waking or occur on waking, as these are classical signs of raised intracranial pressure.

Immediately refer children aged younger than 2 years with any of the following symptoms:
- new-onset seizures
- bulging fontanelle
- extensor attacks
- persistent vomiting.

Urgently or immediately refer children with any of the following neurological symptoms and signs:
- new-onset seizures
- cranial nerve abnormalities
- visual disturbances
- gait abnormalities
- motor or sensory signs
- unexplained deteriorating school performance or developmental mile-stones
- unexplained behavioural and/or mood changes.

Urgent referral
Urgently refer children aged 2 years and older, and young people, with a persistent headache where you cannot carry out an adequate neurological examination in primary care.
Urgently refer children aged younger than 2 years with any of the following symptoms suggestive of CNS cancer:
- abnormal increase in head size
- arrest or regression of motor development
- altered behaviour
- abnormal eye movements, lack of visual following
- poor feeding/failure to thrive.
- squint, urgency dependent on other factors.

Neuroblastoma (all ages)
Urgent referral
Urgently refer children with:
- proptosis
- leg weakness
- unexplained back pain
- unexplained urinary retention.
Investigations
Investigate with a full blood count any of the following symptoms and signs:
- persistent or unexplained bone pain (X-ray also needed)
- pallor
- fatigue
- unexplained irritability
- unexplained fever
- persistent or recurrent upper respiratory tract infections
- generalised lymphadenopathy
- unexplained bruising.
If neuroblastoma is suspected carry out an abdominal examination (and/or urgent ultrasound), and consider chest X-ray and full blood count. If any mass is found, refer urgently.
Infants aged younger than 1 year may have localised abdominal or thoracic masses, and in infants younger than 6 months of age there may also be rapidly progressive intra-abdominal disease. Some babies may present with skin nodules. If any such mass is identified, refer immediately.

Leukaemia (children of all ages)
Immediate referral
Immediately refer children or young people with either unexplained petechiae, or hepatosplenomegaly.

Investigations
Investigate with full blood count and blood film one or more of the following symptoms and signs:
- pallor
- persistent or recurrent upper respiratory tract infections
- fatigue
- generalised lymphadenopathy
- unexplained irritability
- persistent or unexplained bone pain
- unexplained fever
- unexplained bruising.
If the blood film or full blood count indicates leukaemia, make an urgent referral.

Lymphomas
Immediate referral
Immediately refer children or young people with either hepatosplenomegaly, or mediastinal or hilar mass on chest X-ray.

Urgent referral
Urgently refer children or young people with one or more of the following (particularly if there is no evidence of local infection):
- non-tender, firm or hard lymph nodes
- lymph nodes greater than 2 cm in size
- lymph nodes progressively enlarging
- other features of general ill-health, fever or weight loss
- axillary node involvement (in the absence of local infection or dermatitis)
- supraclavicular node involvement
With shortness of breath and unexplained petechiae or hepatosplenomegaly (particularly if not responding to bronchodilators).

Wilms' tumour (all ages)
Wilms' tumour most commonly presents with a painless abdominal mass.
Investigations
Persistent or progressive abdominal distension should prompt abdominal examination:
- if a mass is found, refer immediately.
- if the child or young person is uncooperative and abdominal examination is not possible, consider referral for an urgent abdominal ultrasound.

Urgent referral
Urgently refer a child or young person presenting with haematuria.

Soft tissue sarcoma (all ages)
A soft tissue mass in an unusual location may give rise to misleading local and persistent unexplained symptoms and signs, and sarcoma should be considered. These include:
Head and neck:
- proptosis
- aural polyps/discharge
- persistent unexplained unilateral nasal obstruction with or without discharge and/or bleeding
Genitourinary tract:
- urinary retention
- scrotal swelling
- bloodstained vaginal discharge.
Urgent referral
Urgently refer a child or young person presenting with an unexplained mass at almost any site that has one or more of the following features.
The mass is:
- deep to the fascia
- non-tender
- progressively enlarging
- associated with a regional lymph node that is enlarging
- greater than 2cm in diameter in size.

Bone sarcomas (osteosarcoma and Ewing's sarcoma) (all ages)
Referral
Refer children or young people with:
- rest pain, back pain and unexplained limp (a discussion with a paediatrician or X-ray should be considered before or as well as referral)
- persistent localised bone pain and/or swelling, and X-ray showing signs of cancer. In this case refer urgently.

Retinoblastoma (mostly children less than 2 years)
Urgent referral
Urgently refer children with:
- a white pupillary reflex (leukocoria). Pay attention to parents reporting an odd appearance in their child's eye
- new squint or change in visual acuity if cancer is suspected. (Non-urgently refer if cancer is not suspected.)
- a family history of retinoblastoma and visual problems. (Screening should be offered soon after birth.)

Referral guidelines for suspected cancer

These pages only include the elements of the guidelines that include referral advice. If there is any doubt regarding diagnosis or referral, I recommend you peruse the wealth of extra information in the Quick Reference Guide.

National Institute for Health and Clinical Excellence. *Referral Guidelines for Suspected Cancer: NICE guideline 27*. London: NICE; 2006. Available at: www. nice.org.uk/nicemedia/pdf/CG027quickrefguide.pdf
Reproduced with permission.